A Caregiver's

Love Story

and Reference Guide

Other Books
by Nancie Wiseman Attwater

Teaching Kids to Knit for Martha Stewart Living
Lace from the Attic
Knitted Shawls, Stoles, and Scarves
Knitted Sweaters for Every Season
The Knitter's Book of Finishing Techniques
Classic Knitted Vests
Classic Crochet Vests
Knitting with Wire
Crochet with Wire
The Crochet Book of Finishing Techniques
Start with a Sweatshirt, Book One
Start with a Sweatshirt, Book Two
Jail Journal, Sewing Behind Bars

A Caregiver's

Love Story

and Reference Guide

NANCIE WISEMAN ATTWATER

atmosphere press

Bill,
You are my sun in the morning and my moon at night.
Without you, there would be no story to tell.

Contents

Introduction

Caregiving takes courage, and courage exists when there is fear. Courage allows us to experience freedom and peace. Courage gives us the ability to do something we may be fearful of and keep our wits about us as we do it. Courage is the choice to willingly confront agony, pain, danger, and uncertainty. Courage and caregiving go hand in hand as one person accepts the responsibility for another and their every need.

When caregiving becomes necessary, you do your best with all the love from your heart. It's a job you think you'll never have to do, but when it becomes necessary, you do your best, gathering all your courage to get it right. You may feel your care isn't perfect or how someone else would do it, but you do all you can do, always remembering that your loved one needs you and loves you. This was Bill's life, I was here to make it easier whenever I could, and if I couldn't do it, I would eventually hire help to assist me.

My caregiving was not only physical work but mental work, as well. The worry and wondering about what would happen next was harder than helping Bill. It is in my nature to worry, and now I had extra reasons to wonder what was going on inside Bill. I would wonder what would be next, his blood pressure, thyroid problem, gout, pain, a head injury from a fall? You name it, I would worry about it.

When I was a nurse, I worked ten to twelve hour shifts

in an intensive care unit or the critical care area of a major hospital. What a difference now, from that hard job to my new job hours of 24 hours a day, seven days a week. I was the sole care provider and worrier, with no one to consult. Some days flowed by with no incident, and others seemed to be fraught with issues and problems. Bill and I did our best during these hard times and tried to rest when we needed to, and eat healthy food, and have a laugh or two.

As the first days of illness grew into months and then years and my work increased, never in my wildest dreams did I ever think I would be too busy to run out of the house without combing my hair or putting on lipstick. My friend in Utah I text every day, and I would joke, "Do you know what the back of your hair looks like today?" She had a busy life, too, and would also answer "No" along with me. We had to laugh at this as we were always pretty confident in our dress and our looks when we had the time. Those days were long gone, but I feared they would return sooner rather than later when I would be alone again.

Included in the chapters about taking care of Bill and how we managed the health care system, especially during the pandemic, you'll find information on how to cope with loneliness, aging and cognitive decline, walkers, and wheel-chairs, hiring help, using oxygen, grief, calling an ambulance, taking charge of paperwork, such as medical power of attorney and advance medical directives, and planning to bury your loved one. The last few chapters, includes information that will help you be a loving caregiver, including suggestions for taking care of yourself and how to avoid burnout.

A Caregiver's Love Story is the love story of two people

with very different backgrounds who fell in love and married. It is the story of the fight to keep one alive while the other lives the day-to-day job of caregiving.

Included in each chapter, there is also a lesson - a reward or an idea for you to think about as you read the story of one woman's love for her beloved husband and how she helped him age with grace and live with his terminal illness.

Bill Before Nancie

Lesson: Curiosity, The Beginning of a Brilliant Life

I discovered Bill was probably the single most intelligent person I would ever meet. His knowledge of history made it seem like he had an encyclopedia in his head when he talked about it. Bill was also a huge collector of books and stories about World War Two, as well as memorabilia. More importantly, he was brilliant at his work and every detail that surrounded it.

Bill told me that he used to sit in the backyard of his parent's home at night when he was a young kid and watch the stars and the moon. He would wonder to himself, "Why am I here, who am I?" This seemed unusual to me for a 10-year-old, but it was the beginning of the curiosity of his mind that lead him to a successful lifelong career as an engineer and an attorney. He also was an avid reader and collector of over three thousand lead toy soldiers, many that he painted himself. All done to quell his ever-growing curiosity.

His education was an amazing array of colleges and

degrees. He skipped the 4th grade in grammar school because it was during the Second World War, and he and his parents moved, forcing him to change schools. His grades and intelligence proved to the school that he could easily skip the grade with no problem. And they were right, but in his mind, there was a small issue in that he was a year younger when he graduated high school, and the girls were all older than he was and might not want to go out with him.

Alice, Bill's mother, was his loving companion as he grew up. It was obvious they adored each other. The only time I ever saw Bill cry was when his mother passed away. He was an only child and spent many happy hours with Alice. They cooked together, and he drove her everywhere when he was younger, as she never learned to drive. He would take her to play bridge at her friend's house, and when he picked her up, he would sneak one or two of the leftover little sandwiches that the ladies had eaten for lunch. He considered them his reward for driving.

His father, Bob, was a hardworking man that was away from home for long periods of time, so Alice was taken care of by Bill in his father's absence. They were the best of friends as well as mother and son. She devoured everything he said, laughed at every joke, even if she had heard it before, and took great pride in his job with the state. She would joke, "Bill Attwater is chief counsel of the Water Board, and he has the word "water" in his last name, isn't that funny how that worked out?" Alice was an adorable, loving woman. I was lucky to know her for the short time she was alive after we married.

Bill's parents married on May first; he was born on May second. He loved telling people this and watched for their reaction and then would say, "A year later," and smile mischievously. He loved to joke and then laugh at his own jokes. Sometimes, I would laugh with him, other times I just smiled and let him continue with what he was saying. When Bill doesn't tease or joke with you, you know he isn't feeling well. He doesn't joke much anymore.

In the summer of 1959, Bill's dad asked him to go to Alaska to run one of the gas stations he oversaw. Bill's dad worked for Standard Oil, and they couldn't find anyone willing to go to Alaska. Bill said he would go; he was basically "volunchosen," and his work partner would be Ward, whose dad was the vice president of Standard Oil at the time. This was an adventure of a lifetime, and Bill still tells stories about the experience.

The station was in Mount McKinley National Park, now known as Denali National Park and Preserve. No cars are allowed there now. When Bill was working at the park, cars, trucks, campers, and vans all made their way to his gas station for gas or a tire repair.

Bill was 21, and Ward was not. Bill was able to buy beer at the hotel bar, and they spent the summer reading and talking about everything they could think of when they weren't working or drinking beer. Ward became a history professor in the University of California College system. They still speak. Bill's nickname became "Bugs," and he remains Bugs to this day when he talks to Ward. I am now Mrs. Bugs.

Bill was paid well for his summer in Alaska, and he was then able to pay his tuition to college for an engineering degree. When he graduated, he was commissioned in the Army as a tank officer and was made a first lieutenant. He had been in ROTC in college, so this was a good direction for him to go. His service happened around the time of the Cuban Missile Crisis in the early 1960s.

Before it was time for him to be discharged, he asked his superior officer if he could attend law school if he stayed near enough to the Army base to get there if needed. He was stationed at Fort Lewis, Washington. Permission was granted, and he attended law school at the University of Washington in Seattle, where he finished his law degree seven months early. He graduated early instead of doing Law Review, as his professors suggested he do. He was nervous the whole time he was in school because he thought he might have to return to the Army, and it would interrupt his education. Fortunately, he was never called back to the base and was eventually given an honorable discharge.

Bill moved to Sacramento, California, and took a job as a senior attorney with the Department of Water Resources. After a few years, The Water Resources Control Board was formed, and he transferred there and was asked to be chief counsel. He was appointed by then-governor Ronald Reagan. Bill would remain in this job for over thirty years. This was unusual because when new governors are elected, they often replace some of their most important positions with members of their own party. Bill remained in his job through Democratic and Republican governors without an issue.

Bill signed hundreds of thousands of documents that are in the state archives as - @ or @H20 for Attwater. His secretary even had a rubber stamp made for him with the @ symbol. He continues to use the symbol to this day instead of his initials. No one ever had an issue with this, and everyone seemed to know what and who it meant. This was long before email and the frequent use of the @ symbol, as we know it now.

Bill went to the United States Supreme Court representing the state of California twice during his time as chief counsel. He became the expert on Proposition 65 and traveled around the United States, informing businesses in other states what the proposition was about and what it would mean to them if they chose to do business in California. This is the proposition that forced businesses to label their products for the possibility of causing cancer, congenital defects, or reproductive harm. It also prohibits California businesses from knowingly discharging significant amounts of listed toxins into drinking water.

After over thirty years as chief counsel, Bill retired over twenty years ago. He can still tell stories of his work, like Clint Eastwood showing up at his office one day, and give you his grades from law school. He has no problem citing the laws from his work of many years ago. His current memories fail him now, and operating the remote control for the TV is a problem, but he still has a very active mind.

During Bill's early years as chief counsel, he was married to his first wife, who helped him raise three children, two adopted and one theirs, as well as taking care of his aging parents. Their divorce was amicable and what seemed fair and equitable to me. Their reason for divorcing, apparently, was because they grew apart. Bill was the up-and-coming executive for the state of California, and she could not relate to his work or his need for travel. I believe the kids, all three are over 50 years old, so not really "kids," are still angry at him over the divorce.

Bill's youngest daughter was a gymnast, and he took her to lessons many evenings while doing his very important job for the state. His oldest daughter was a soccer player, and Bill became the referee for her soccer games. His son was in trouble often, and he was eventually asked to leave the house by his mother. He would remain distant for the rest of his life.

None of the kids ever warmed up to me. I tried for years, and one day, Bill told me, "Give up, they've hated you since the day I married you." I was heartbroken, but then I didn't know how to be a stepmom either. I shed many a tear over these children and my inability to understand them or get along with them.

Whenever Bill had a medical emergency, I would call his oldest daughter and she would let her siblings know what was happening. We used the phrase, "dumb it down" for his youngest daughter because she didn't seem to understand what it meant to have a medical emergency. I gave up trying to talk to her and let her sister deal with her. Yet, she seemed to have some curiosity about the possibility of an inheritance as she asked for a copy of the Will recently. Bill told her "No."

Bill's son was always a problem. I never spoke to him as it always ended in a screaming match followed by horrible emails. Both girls quit visiting years ago except for maybe once or twice a year. They live thirty minutes away.

When the kids were young, Bill spent time helping them with homework and kept them busy with sports and a big swimming pool he had installed in their back yard. He loved being the referee for his oldest daughter's soccer games and enjoyed going to the games with her. At one of the games, he tripped in a hole on the soccer field and twisted his ankle. He thought it was sprained and limped around for weeks on it without going to the doctor. He has always been too busy to go to the doctor, it seems.

Thirty-some plus years later, he would find out that the ankle had been broken and did not heal correctly. He always walked with a bit of a limp, and then he would frequently have gout that would attack the same foot, and he would lay down in agony until the pain went away. Cortisone shots and compression socks helped the pain for a while, but he eventually gave all of it up and started using a cane. He now uses a walker and can barely walk without help.

Bill never complained about his ankle but would always walk with a limp. He frequently walked from his office to the capital just a few blocks away or out to lunch with some of his work friends. Sometimes I would meet him at his office before I opened my shop to have coffee with him, and we would walk to a local coffee shop without a word from Bill about pain. I could see his limp was getting worse over time. Walking would become a major issue for Bill, and eventually, getting out of a chair would become a problem. He is in bed now more than he is out but will always dress and come to the kitchen for his meals and to read the newspapers he loves.

Bill continued to decline as the years passed, but his spirit was always a central figure in the room. As dementia and lung disease started to affect his brain, he would be at a loss for words and recent memories sometimes. This was difficult for him when he could not remember a word and would look to me for help. Losing his independence would be one of the hardest things for him to grapple with, but he did it with a smile on his face and tried to remember his wonderful life the best he could.

Bill's life was a gift not only for me but the environment and his co-workers. He has had many experiences that few will ever have. His life seemed to glow from the beginning, and with some help now, it will continue for as long as possible to be full of learning, reading, and his never-ending curiosity. He remains a happy individual despite the many diseases and illnesses that seem to plague him.

Nancie Before Bill

Lesson: Practice Gratefulness Whenever Faced with Adversity

My life growing up was the opposite of Bills. I had two older brothers, six and twelve years older than me. I adored them. They were what felt like the only sane thing in the household where I grew up. Charlie, six years older, babysat me and entertained me while my mother worked in the evenings. He kept life as normal as possible for us, which was difficult when my mother wasn't around much. When both brothers left the house at eighteen to join the military, I was devastated. I was now alone while my mother worked in the evenings to support us.

My father had passed away when I was 4, and I don't believe my mother ever recovered from his death. She was left to care for the three of us on her own with little support from her family. There were days we didn't have enough to eat, but no one seemed to care. She went to work in the evenings to earn more money than our Social Security

Survivor's Benefits provided to keep us clothed and fed, but it was a struggle. She was depressed all her life, and, I believe, angry at the world because of what happened to her when my dad passed away. I don't think she ever forgave him for dying.

She had many boyfriends, but no one seemed to stick around for long, and frankly, that was okay with me. They disrupted the little bit of normal that we had in our house. My brothers didn't know many of them as they were gone, but they knew the situation was not great for me, and there was just nothing much they could do about it. They were young and trying to create a life for themselves that did not include my mother, and it seemed me.

One of my fondest memories of childhood, and probably the only one, is that my brothers came up with the idea of my "half-birthday." I was born June 25th, making December 25th my half-birthday. Once they figured this out, it became their goal to make it special. On Christmas, I would get half of a present and the other half on my birthday. They were always wrapped in birthday wrapping paper. It could have been half a set of crayons, a puzzle with half the pieces missing, or even a pair of pajamas with only the top, not the bottoms, or vice versa. My brother to this day calls Christmas Nancie's half-birthday, not Christmas.

We were never a family that said, "I love you." We still don't. My youngest brother is terminally ill with lung cancer now, and occasionally one of us will quietly utter the words, but it does not come easily. My older brother passed away over thirty years ago from lung cancer, the same as my dad.

After the boys left and my mother continued to work in the evenings, I was left alone in the house. I call myself the "original latchkey kid," as it was not common in the sixties for a child to come home to an empty house after school. I would do my homework and watch TV, but mostly I sewed. My mother was a seamstress when she wasn't working, and I helped her with some of her sewing for her customers. This, I believe, saved me and gave me a career in needlework and many happy hours by myself.

Eventually, I would graduate from high school and want to go to college. The money my mother received from Social Security was supposed to have been saved for me to go to school and would continue if I was in college full-time until age twenty-two. She promised me I would be able to go to college, but when it came down to paying for it, there was nothing in the savings account. I don't believe she ever thought I would make it to college, so she didn't make any effort to support the idea.

My oldest brother invited me to live with him, his wife, and small daughter in a town seventy-five miles away from my mother. I was to help with the house and babysit my niece while going to school and working. I was thrilled about this and left my mother's house when I turned eighteen. I had been working part-time while in high school in a pizza restaurant and saved enough money to buy a car and get out of the house. I called it my "escape" money.

All was good at my brother's house for about eight months when my sister-in-law announced that the situation wasn't working for her anymore. To this day, I'm not sure what she was mad about. She told my brother to kick me out of the house. I had to quit college, go to work full-time, and find an apartment. I was eighteen years old and on my own.

My full-time job was at a fabric store. My sewing

knowledge really paid off here, and it was how I got the job in the first place. One day a customer came into the store looking for someone to make her daughter's wedding gown and three bridesmaid's dresses. The manager recommended me. I had not done that elaborate kind of sewing, but I was willing to try, as this could mean a lot of money so I could go back to school. It was a brave step because I could have ruined a lot of expensive fabric. Thankfully the dresses turned out beautiful, and I was allowed to attend the wedding so I could see the bride walk down the aisle in my creation.

I saved enough money to get back into college in the fall of the next year. This time it was a four-year college instead of the community college I had been attending. I lived in the dorm and was thrilled to be back in school like all my friends from high school, who by now were sophomores. I was still a freshman but didn't care. While attending college, I drove thirty minutes to work at the same fabric store I had been working at while I was out of school. I worked about 16 hours a week in the evenings and weekends. I did this for about two years and then my car fell apart, and I could only afford a small motorcycle to get around on. I would eventually find a job near the campus and my dorm.

I spent the next Christmas with the family I had made the wedding dresses for because I could not go home. One day the mother said to me, "Why are you working so much, when you are getting your Social Security?" I responded, "What Social Security?" She explained that I should be getting a monthly check to help pay for college from Social Security because of my dad's death when I was young.

I didn't know anything about this, so I called the Social

Security office, and it was explained to me that my mother was getting my checks. I couldn't believe how mean this was of her. I told them to change the address to mine and never told my mom. I started getting the checks, and she figured out what I had done and quit talking to me for several years. She was making her car payment with my checks—I was riding a small motorcycle because I couldn't afford a car.

I finished nursing school and moved to Sacramento, where I found a great job at a local hospital. I loved the work, and the hospital was a wonderful step up for me. I worked in Renal Dialysis and eventually the Intensive Care Unit, where I took care of open-heart surgery and critically ill patients. I worked there for about twenty years.

After about fifteen years as a nurse, I opened a yarn store. I always wanted to own one, and the opportunity just fell into place. I was an avid knitter and loved sewing and quilting. A local quilt store wanted to move to a larger store and asked me if I wanted to share space with them, as they knew my desire to open a yarn store. I jumped at the chance and opened my little part of the store while I still worked full-time at the hospital. By this time, I had bought a house and still needed to keep the payments up and also subsidize the shop while it was getting started.

Eventually, I would move out of the shared space into a shop of my own in a strip mall not far from the original location. It was also right across the street from the ice cream shop that Bill would eventually visit and see my sign across the street in the window that would bring him into my store. The sign said, "Sweater Repair."

My shop thrived for twelve years. After we were married, Bill helped me in numerous ways. He cooked and served meals for special events we hosted, and I had the freedom to travel and teach all over the country. We made knitting videos and named our production company "Wisewater Productions," combining our two names into one. I can't tell you how many of those videos we sold, but it was an overwhelming amount when I think back on it. My shop was called "Nancie Knits," and Bill was called "Mr. Knits" by many of my customers who knew and loved him. He never blinked an eye at this as I think he enjoyed talking to my customers and helping me.

I was gone many weekends teaching at conventions and for local knitting guilds. Bill was so patient about this and never complained. He stayed home and took care of the dogs, or if I was going somewhere wonderful like Charleston, South Carolina or Clearwater, Florida he went with me. I worked, and he went sightseeing. It was a glorious time for us both.

I wrote my first book during this time as well. I would not have been able to do this if it had not been for Bill taking care of everything from the shopping to the laundry and the cooking. I was pampered beyond belief, and many people were jealous of his cooking dinner and taking care of the yard and house, not to mention the dogs and me. I knew I was lucky, but little did I know just how much work this had been for him until I had to start taking care of all these duties myself.

My life changed completely after we were married, from a family I never saw to having a loving husband who cared about me deeply. I learned to "love" someone, something I never learned as a kid, and it is difficult to give love when you have never been shown love. I always wondered how I was so lucky that Bill would want to marry and take care of me. I still marvel at this over twenty-eight years later.

We Begin

Lesson: Trust Each Other for Understanding and Strength When All Around You Appears Chaotic

We lived in a retirement community where many of the residents had been married for over fifty years. We just celebrated our twenty-ninth anniversary and I think some of our neighbors would have considered us newlyweds. Our lives had changed dramatically after our chance meeting and then marriage. As with any marriage, there would be many transitions over the years that made an immense difference in our relationship. The caregiver role and the responsibilities of running the household would also change as they frequently do when one or both marriage partners have aged or experienced poor health. This is our love story.

While I owned my yarn store in Sacramento for twelve years, I also worked as a registered nurse in a local hospital. Bill walked into my store in the spring of 1992 with a yellow cotton sweater that had a hole in the shoulder seam that needed to be repaired. He frequented the ice cream shop across the street and had seen my sign on the front window of my shop that read, "Sweater Repair."

He was wearing a beautiful suit and tie and was apparently on his lunch hour from his work in downtown Sacramento. I would later learn his office was near the capital. We had a nice chat. I looked at his sweater and told him when the repair would be finished and the cost. He didn't leave as most men coming into a yarn store would since they are a bit uncomfortable there. Instead, he stayed and talked with a favorite customer of mine who was sitting at the table knitting. I got busy, and he eventually went on his way. But before he left, he gave me his business card. This was no ordinary guy - he was Chief Counsel for the State of California Water Resources Control Board. I was impressed, a lawyer, a nice man, handsome, and very friendly.

It seemed he had a lot of sweaters that needed repairs; or had friends that needed sweater repairs because he kept coming back. I didn't think too much about it, but the customer who had a nice chat with him on the first day said to me, "You don't get it, do you?" "What, get what?" I asked. She said, "He keeps coming back to see you so he can talk to you." I just laughed and walked away. But it did make me think.

On his subsequent visits, we had several conversations, both thinking the other was married. But when each of us spoke of the "we" in our life, it was about our dogs, not our spouses. Finally, when this was all figured out, and the conversations were getting more personal, he came in one Saturday while eating an ice cream cone he purchased at the store across the street. He had been riding his bike and lived in the area, so stopped for an ice cream cone, but I believe he had another plan to visit me. Maybe he was getting his courage up.

Again, he was very friendly. We chatted some more, but it was just about closing time, and I was wondering to myself, "How am I going to get him to leave?" I needed to get home and rest because I was working at the hospital that night. I think he sensed this, and the conversation sped up a bit, and he eventually asked me if I wanted to go to lunch. I was surprised and didn't quite know how to handle his invitation. I explained, "I can't leave for lunch during the week as I don't have an employee to take over the store, but maybe on the weekend"?

He suggested we go the next day, a Sunday. Again, I had to explain. "I work the 11 p.m. to 7 a.m. shift tonight at the hospital and need to sleep part of Sunday, but maybe a quick bite after I get up would work." He agreed that would be perfect, and we set up a time.

The next day, Sunday, I got up and dressed in a pants and jacket outfit. I didn't know where we were going and thought I better dress nicely because of who I was going out with. I was wrong, of course, because he was in a casual outfit, and I was overdressed. It didn't seem to matter, and I don't think he noticed. We went out for Japanese food, which we both loved, and spent a couple of hours talking and getting to know each other better.

Bill continued to drop by the shop frequently for a visit or to make a dinner invitation, and I was beginning to see this might become serious. Then, I got scared and nervous. I had never dated much and didn't know "the rules," so to speak, and he was such an important guy. I wasn't sure I was up to his standards. It was obvious he was very intelligent. Was I going to be able to keep up with him?

A couple of weeks later, he flew to Los Angeles on

business, and before his return flight home, he called to see if I was interested in going to dinner that night. I accepted but was nervous. This was happening very fast, in my mind. There was clearly an age difference between us, but it didn't seem to make a difference when we were together.

We went to dinner, and I tried to explain that I was not used to dating and I needed to slow down a little bit, as I was getting very nervous about the speed our relationship was moving. I was forty-one and had never been married! He was very understanding, and the evening ended on a happy note.

A few days later, I received a lovely letter in the mail, that Bill had handwritten. He wanted to reassure me that he was just a regular guy that cooked, cleaned, did his laundry, and just wanted my company because he liked me. I was so taken with this letter that I called him and told him I would continue to go out with him, but because of my work schedule, it could not be as frequently as he might like.

About a month later, it was Bill's birthday. I had to work at the hospital until 7 p.m. that day, but he invited me to dinner after my work shift was over. Normally, he was an early eater, so I knew this was going to be a sacrifice for him. When I arrived, he had a nice dinner prepared, and we ate out on the patio. It was the first time I had been to his home. He showed me around and introduced me to his dog, Polly.

He asked me to spend the night, but I explained I had to get home to my dog and would need some clothing for the next day because we were planning to take a ride to Napa to have lunch and wander the shops. He suggested, "I can take you home to get your clothes and toiletries." I said, "No, I'll go alone, I'll be quick." "I also need to bring the dog back with me or I can't stay." "No problem, bring the dog," he said, and I was off to gather what I needed.

The next day was lovely. Lunch was fabulous, and we went to some of the local shops. I realized that Bill might be as nervous as I was. We were in a glass and dish shop where he knocked down a whole rack of items, fortunately not glass. I don't think he was clumsy, he was just trying to impress me, and this rack got in his way. We still laugh about it.

I began spending more and more time with him at his home. He would go to my house and get my mail and my dog. Often my dog, Christina, stayed at his house with Polly, or I took her to work with me. We were falling into a lovely pattern of dinners and evenings together. I didn't know how to cook very well because I always worked evenings at the hospital and ate dinner there, so he did all of the cooking. Our quiet time after dinner was spent watching TV or sitting on the patio talking.

We began to take weekend trips to the coast, enjoying the beach and the sunsets or the mountains. They were wonderful trips, full of sightseeing and long car rides where we would talk about everything in our lives that was going on or what we had done in the past. This was when we got to know each other. I would hang a sign in my shop window that said, "Gone Fishing," if I closed on a Saturday so we could spend more time away.

I would always be knitting when we were together because I needed to keep up with samples for the shop, and it was how I spent my time when I wasn't working, but I worked a lot! I continued to work at the hospital on a part-time basis as well as running my shop. Bill was very patient about all of this, as I was with his toy soldier collection that he spent many hours painting and researching. Eventually, over a few months, all my things were moved to his house, and it seemed I had moved in with him. My small house became a rental, and I would eventually sell it.

About six months after we met, Bill asked me, "Does our age difference matter to you?" He was fifty-three, and I was forty-one. I didn't think it did. In fact, I told him, "I barely notice it except you are far more experienced and educated than I am." He told me not to worry. We became engaged and married just a little over a year after we met. Bill wanted to marry sooner, but since I was so unsure of myself and being married, I asked that we live together for about a year. I had no health insurance, and he desperately wanted to get me on his policy. But I was stubborn and wanted to wait.

We had a simple wedding in the backyard of his/our house. It was intimate and heartwarming as both of our mothers were still alive to attend, my brother and sister-in-law were there, as well as Bill's three adult children, along with a handful of friends. The two dogs stayed at the dog sitter's home, or they would have been there too.

Bill wrote our wedding vows. Very simple and very sweet even after all these years.

"Nancie and Bill have come together in mid-life. Each has spent many years maturing into the individuals that they are today. Each has educated themselves in professions and the ways of the world. Each has contributed to the betterment of this world in their own way; either by helping the sick, inspiring creativity, or by protecting the environment. Each are suited to the other. Each has found in the other goodness, tenderness, and happiness. Each has promised to help each other in every way they can. Nancie and Bill love each other with a tenderness and goodness that will make this world a better place. Nancie and Bill have pledged to be honest with each other and will trust each other for understanding and strength when all around them appears chaotic."

These words were appropriate then, and even more so now. There was no need for the common phrase "in sickness and in health." That was understood from the start, without question. We still live by those words.

Our decorations were very basic, made by me. There were a few flowers, and I put together a white arch and decorated it in the backyard, so we had a lovely place to stand to say our vows. Bill fixed all of the food for the guests, and a friend picked up the cake for us to share with everyone. We left for our honeymoon that evening, and since I had not eaten anything at the reception, we stopped at Arby's, one of my favorite places for fast food. Not a very fancy place to eat, but it brings back fond memories of our special day every time we see one.

Our hotel at Bodega Bay was on the beach where we stayed for one night, and then we drove to San Francisco to embark on our first cruise together. We went to Alaska, where Bill had worked when he was younger. This would be the first of many cruises for us as our wonderful life began together.

The day before every anniversary, we joke about the arch. One of us will say, "Is the arch still up and decorated, or did the wind blow it down yet?" There was a gentle breeze the day of the wedding, and you could see the arch sway with it. We held our breath that it would stay up.

In our minds, for every anniversary that arch still sways a bit in the wind as we remember the lovely day with friends and family.

The yellow sweater Bill brought in on the first day I met him remains in my closet next to my wedding dress. It's very faded and almost white. I found it very comforting to wear when I traveled, or he did. I felt he was close if I had the sweater on. I take it out and look at it every now and then. I always smile at the memories it conjures of those nervous days when Bill was courting me.

Our Life Together

Lesson: Travel Before it's Too Late

After our honeymoon cruise, Bill fell in love with cruising just as I had after my first cruise. We took many wonderful trips through the Panama Canal, around Australia, New Zealand, and the Caribbean. We then began to travel to England and France. These were perfect places for Bill as the World War II landmarks were a trip back in history for him. He loved touring the D-day beaches in France and the museums in England. I loved them too, and I was beginning to enjoy the history as much as he did. We also went to art galleries and many other museums, but much of our time was spent going to the sites where famous battles took place.

We spent many happy days learning more about each other - our likes and dislikes as well as our little quirks. Bill loved to cook, he would shop on the way home from work, and when I got home, dinner was ready and handed to me. He had gone to cooking school in San Francisco and loved all the pots, pans, and toys that went along with it. He tells people I could barely boil water when we married, which wasn't quite true, but close.

We both still worked at this time. I had my shop, and Bill continued work as chief counsel. I took Friday and Sunday off, and he took Saturday and Sunday off, so we had Sunday together to catch up and rest. The schedule worked quite well for both of us. I also began teaching knitting all over the United States at conventions and seminars, and I began to travel quite a bit. Often, I was gone every other weekend. By this time, I had a great employee who took care of the shop for me. I was so confident in her that I was comfortable leaving for long weekends. Bill went with me occasionally, so it became time off for him to travel, too.

I wrote my first book during this time. A customer gave me a handwritten notebook from the late 1800's with little, tiny samples of knitted lace sewn to the page with the directions. It had been found in the trash of a Victorian Home in downtown Sacramento when it was being cleaned out. I spent months researching the author of the notebook and her special abbreviations for knitted lace. This book became the first of 14 books I would write. I began to love writing books as much as I enjoyed knitting and teaching knitting.

About seven years after we were married, Bill decided to retire. He was 62, and I was surprised because I thought he would work until he was at least 65. The office staff had a lovely retirement party for him, with over one hundred people in attendance. It was heartwarming to hear all the wonderful things his co-workers said about him and his career.

Coincidentally, at the time of his retirement, I was invited to teach in Washington state at the Coupeville Art Center on Whidbey Island. Bill traveled with me on this trip, as he was familiar with the area, having gone to law school in Seattle. While I was teaching, he roamed around the Island and found a three-story house for sale on the beach. The house faced the Straits of Juan de Fuca and Canada. He came to get me out of class so I could see it, too. It was gorgeous, and the view was unsurpassed by any house in the area.

We flew home and talked about buying the house while in the air. I commented, "We can always come back to Sacramento if it doesn't work out, but let's not grow old wishing we had moved to the beach and never followed through with the dream." One of our concerns was that it was a three-story, four thousand square foot house. It was huge.

The next day, Bill went to work, and I was instructed to call and make an offer on the house. Three days later, we had purchased the house and were going to put our house in Sacramento up for sale. We had no intention of moving when Bill retired, but I had closed my shop the year before, thinking that Bill would retire soon, and we might travel more. It was a good decision.

It was a whirlwind move. We bought the house in early April and moved to Washington in early June. We packed everything we could fit in a U-Haul truck, and the movers were going to take everything else. We had three dogs when we moved, our golden retriever rode with Bill in the truck, and I had the two little dogs in my VW Bug as we headed north to Washington. It took us two days to get there. I had never driven that far and was amazed at how well we managed going so far with our three dogs.

Whidbey Island is about thirty-seven miles long and one

to ten miles wide, depending on what part of the Island you're on. It's shaped a bit like a crescent and at the very top, or northern end, is the small town of Oak Harbor, where a naval base is located. Our home was on the curve of the Island, pointing out to sea. The Island was only about two miles wide at this point, and I could walk from edge to edge in just a short time.

To get to the Island, which is about thirty miles off the coast of the mainland of Washington, we had to ride a car ferry. It was only a thirty-minute trip, but it was a huge shift from the hustle and bustle of city life to the beautiful, quiet life of living on the beach and watching the ocean. We could feel our pulse calm and our breathing quiet as the Island came into view from the ferry.

The house was another forty-five minutes from the ferry, driving through gorgeous forests and a few small towns. We could see water on both sides of the island as we drove the two-lane road that traversed the entire length of the island. One lane going in, and one going out. If the traffic got snarled for some reason, all traffic came to a halt. There was no alternative route.

We soon settled in and began our life on "Island Time." That's what living on an island is like being in a different time zone from the rest of the world. If you called someone to do work on your house, they might show up, and they might not, as everyone follows the relaxed feel of living on an island. There was a small hospital, grocery shopping, and even a Starbucks on the island, so it wasn't necessary to leave very often unless you needed a big shopping trip for clothes, food, a major appliance, or a large hospital for a specialty doctor.

We did leave the Island once a month or so, but not in the winter, as the weather could get pretty terrible with gale-force winds. To get to the airport in Seattle, it was at least a two-and-a-half-hour drive as long as you didn't miss the ferry. During the summer, the ferry line would back up for hours due to the tourists wanting to visit. You could be in line for two hours or more, waiting for the thirty-minute ferry ride unless you left very early in the morning.

We settled into island life and the easy flow of day-to-day life rather quickly until winter began to set in. Bill knew what would happen with the weather since he lived in the area when he was younger, but I was ill-prepared for the weather and the darkness. The back of our house faced the Straits of Juan de Fuca, which is the shipping lane out of Puget Sound to the Pacific Ocean, and it was a wind tunnel!

We could get winds up to sixty-five miles per hour frequently. It rattled the house and sounded like a freight train rolling through the master bedroom located on the third floor. I still do not like wind. I hate wind! I would move to the lower bedroom with the dogs and try to get away from the noise. The golden retriever was terrified, too, and would try and get between the box spring and the mattress to escape the noise.

The Island was so far north that it would get dark at 4:00 p.m. and not get light until 9:00 a.m. in the winter, but in the summer, it would get light at 5:00 a.m. and stay light until 10:00 p.m. This took some adjusting, and so did the temperature drop in the winter, which was very cold for me. We also got snow and a fair amount of rain, which I didn't mind. It was the wind that tortured me, but Bill didn't mind any of it.

I found the depression that I had managed well in California was aggravated by the weather and the cold in Washington. Even though I was still traveling and teaching, and was able to leave now and then, it just wasn't enough for me. I also had constant migraine headaches because of the barometric pressure changes that occurred while I was basically living in the middle of an ocean.

We had large windows on the side of the house facing the beach and the ocean that allowed us to see mother nature at her best. An eagle lived in a tree just a short distance from our deck. Orca whales went past our beach as they migrated north or south, depending on the season. We also had a great white whale or two go by occasionally. Cruise ships would pass by just close enough that you wanted to wave to the people on board. The Navy also flew helicopters along the coast, and one day it looked like one was going to land on our deck. They were that close!

A few years after our move to the Island, serious health problems would plague both Bill and me. I fell and fractured my back, and had a couple of surgeries for gallstones, and acid reflux. But these were minor, compared to Bill. He developed an aneurysm in his right groin that needed to be taken care of. We went to a doctor in Everett, Washington, to discuss the surgery. The aneurysm was in a major artery that fed the leg, and it was a very dangerous surgery because of the potential for bleeding.

Bill was admitted to the hospital in Everett, which by the way, wasn't much closer than Seattle and still required the ferry ride to get there. I took him to the hospital and would stay in a nearby hotel, so I didn't have to drive back and forth to visit and then pick him up to come home. I was a nervous wreck for this surgery. My ICU nurse training told me that this would not be life-threatening, but when it's your husband, the rules don't always make sense. I anxiously waited for him to get out of surgery and admitted to the intensive care unit of the hospital.

Bill did great and was discharged in a couple of days. On the way home, after the ferry ride, he got nauseated. Bill was always the driver, not the passenger, and was prone to get car sick. I called the doctor from the car and got some nausea medicine prescribed, so I could pick it up on the way home from the pharmacy in town. He was better when he got home and took the medicine, but then the recovery process started. It was a painful surgery, and when Bill doesn't feel well, he goes to bed and sleeps. Long, long naps and sleeping all night are his cure.

He was continuing to do all the cooking when we were on the Island, and with him resting and recovering, I took over making the little bit I could fix that appealed to him. Thankfully this didn't go on too long because I was running out of recipes that I knew how to prepare. Bill was soon back on his feet again, but the ankle problem was beginning to get worse, so the two sets of stairs in the house were becoming difficult to manage, along with the pain from his incision. Bill lived mostly on the second floor of the house where the kitchen, a bedroom, and bathroom were located.

This surgery was the beginning of small health issues that seemed to add together to make it harder and harder for Bill to get around. He began driving again and did the shopping, but he no longer walked the golden retriever, as the hills were becoming difficult for him, and he needed to rest more.

Bill's old ankle injury began to give him more pain while we were on the Island as well. He wore heavy boots to keep his ankle supported, and that seemed to work quite well. We walked the streets of London and Paris while he wore those boots, but the limp and shuffle of his foot were getting more pronounced. He slipped off a curb in London and twisted his bad ankle, and that sent him to bed to rest before we could continue with our trip.

I began to take over some of the responsibilities of our travel. When we rented a car, I did the driving. I drove from the outlying area of Paris into the airport in a very fast little Saab car. The traffic was crazy, and thankfully, Bill read the map and kept me in the right lanes so we didn't get lost and miss our flight home.

Gout would often attack Bill's already painful right ankle, and he would take a drug called Colchicine to stop the pain. This medicine works, but it must be taken until you get diarrhea, and then the pain will go away. The cure was often worse than the illness in this respect. I learned it was best to watch from the hallway as he slept in bed. It was better not to disturb him, even though my medical background told me there had to be a better way to treat this problem. I would find out eventually that there really is no alternative to treat gout, but diet can prevent it.

Gout has long been known as the "disease of kings" because of the lavish diet and alcohol consumption of the wealthy, like King Henry VIII, who suffered from it. In Bill's case, diet didn't seem to change things. He was diagnosed with gout at a very early age and did not eat the foods that normally exacerbate it. Gout in the same ankle that he had injured was so intolerable he had to keep his foot up and wait for the pain to pass. I tried to manage the house and dogs while he recovered, but this was becoming more and more frequent, and harder for Bill to deal with. He developed a very pronounced limp and would use a cane when the pain was too much.

During this time, I had several surgeries and fell and fractured a vertebra in my back. Bill took care of me, bringing me food and taking me to the doctor. I slept in the bedroom on the third floor, and the stairs were becoming an issue for me, too. I recovered, but I lost a lot of weight and did not look well.

I continued to write books, but I had to quit traveling, or I would never recover. This change was sad for both of us since Bill used to go with me on some of my trips. Our happy marriage was feeling the strain of both of us having some health issues, and finally, when I could no longer walk due to back pain and used a wheelchair, I begged Bill to move back to our old area in Sacramento for both medical care and a one-story house.

Bill was not happy leaving his beautiful home on the beach, but I saw no other way for us to continue living there. We went to Palm Springs to get out of the cold that winter, and I did nothing but sleep. I was sad, depressed, and in pain. He finally suggested that we move back to California, even though he really did not want to. If we did not love each other so much, I felt this could have been the end of our marriage. I thought I would have to leave the Island by myself.

We flew down to Sacramento and spent a week looking for our new home. We were moving from our very large house to a smaller one-story home. We were lucky and found a large home with huge rooms for all the cabinets and books we had, plus a sewing room and an office for me. We looked at several houses, but this was our first choice, and we were lucky enough to purchase it.

I injured my back again while looking for our new home and was in agony for months. Nothing helped, and the small hospital and physical therapy department on the Island could not do much for me. Nothing I did would make it better. I just had to lay down. This meant Bill did the packing. It was difficult to watch, but I could not do anything.

Driving my car back to California because of my back injury would have been impossible, so I flew down, and Bill and the dogs drove down a few days later. We shipped my car, and Bill hired someone to help him make the long drive. I was not much help, and I knew it and feel bad about it to this day. Bill had to do all the work and leave his beloved house on the beach.

The moving van arrived a few days later, and we began to settle in and learn about our new neighborhood. We were used to the weather here, so there were no surprises since the new house was about forty-five minutes from our old house in Sacramento. We moved to a Del Webb community, which is an over fifty-five adult community that has all the amenities of a cruise ship on land. The gardens are maintained beautifully, and two golf courses snake their way through the houses. It's green all year here.

I believe the move saved us both. Finally, I found a doctor with our new health insurance that got me into the right physical therapist, and I eventually recovered from my back injury. It was a long, hard recovery, but finally, I was able to walk without pain. I never thought I would get better. Bill's life was saved, too, as he began to have heart and lung problems and more issues with walking. In the end, I believe it saved our marriage too.

We were happy, and it seemed we made a good decision in moving back to California. Our new home was beautiful, the area was lovely, and the neighbors were friendly. We both began to feel well again, and it looked like our life was on the right track. Bill volunteered for a couple of committees at the lodge, and I began to teach again. Things were moving in the right direction for us both. But just when we thought we were on the right track with our health, new problems popped up for both of us. But then, life can be tricky and creep up on you sometimes, and before you know it, it's made a left turn instead of a right.

Bill would have many more surgeries and get much weaker, and I would eventually be diagnosed with Lupus and Rheumatoid Arthritis, which can lead to devastating illnesses and joint deformities. I was given several medications to try and fight off the symptoms and eventually started a chemotherapy-type drug that was infused every month at the hospital. I felt well or maybe just well enough to function, most of the time, but the fatigue could often be overwhelming. Many times, when Bill laid down in the afternoon for a nap, I would lay down too. If he was not up and moving around, I felt it was a good time for me to rest, too.

Surgery and the Fall in the Hall

Lesson: You Never Know How Strong You Are Until it is Your Only Choice

A few years after we moved, Bill began having trouble with the aneurysm that had been repaired in Washington. A CT scan showed that the aneurysm was growing, and the first repair had not held. He saw a vascular surgeon, and surgery was scheduled for ten days later. It would be a major surgery, and he would stay a few nights in the hospital. The surgery would be long, and I expected it to be a long recovery, too. Bill would need a lot of care at home.

Bill had the surgery, and spent five days in the hospital. This was a much more extensive surgery than the previous one, with one incision on each groin, to place a Y-shaped tubing in his aorta and femoral arteries. The six-hour surgery was finished, but after several hours in the recovery room, there was talk of the possibility of taking him back to surgery because of a "leak" in the repair, but fortunately, that did not have to happen.

The incisions were very painful, and standing and walking were difficult. The doctor wanted to send him to a skilled nursing facility, but I refused and said I would take care of him at home. I picked him up at the hospital, we came home, and he went to bed. He was on strong pain medicine, and the best place for him was tucked in bed. He tried to get up for meals, which, believe me, weren't much, but he was doing his best to eat a little each day.

My hypervigilance kicked in, and my plan for taking care of Bill was to try and think of what "might" happen before it happened. If I stayed on top of his needs, made sure he drank liquids and ate a little something each day, I knew he would get well.

His incisions did not heal well, and he needed dressing changes frequently. A nurse came to see him once, and then I took over from there. The dressing changes weren't difficult, but annoying for Bill to have to have it done. He wanted to do it himself, which is in his nature. This was, of course, impossible because he couldn't even see the incisions. He didn't want to bother me.

He was recovering nicely but slowly. I tried to cook things he liked to eat and help him get around the house. He had a walker, but it did not have wheels, and he hated it. It was the typical silver metal walker used in the hospital. It was clunky, he thought, and too hard to push around, so he didn't use it much. He was just not ready to be dependent on a walker. He wanted to use me instead. I would hold his hand as he walked and try to keep him balanced, but he is quite a bit taller and heavier than me, and this was not the best solution.

His primary care doctor at this time was really a putz, to

put it bluntly. He wrote prescriptions for pain medicine like it was candy without even seeing Bill. I was concerned Bill was getting used to taking the pills and liked them a lot because they let him sleep rather than try and do some walking and get his strength back. I don't think he ever really got addicted to them, but it did affect his judgment and ability to walk. I quit filling the prescriptions and eventually put him on plain Tylenol, and this basically "woke him up."

Three weeks after the surgery, Bill got up to get a glass of milk in the middle of the night. On the way back to the bedroom, he fell. I heard this loud thud and then a crash. He tried to hold the glass of milk up, so it didn't hit the floor, and get broken, rather than trying to block his fall with his hands. He ended up falling flat on his face and his left knee. This was a dead heap fall right on his nose.

He cut his nose at the bridge where his glasses would rest and was bleeding profusely when I found him just a few seconds later. As I ran for the phone, I grabbed some ice to put on his nose, and then I called an ambulance. They arrived quickly, got him on the gurney, and took him to the hospital. I feared he had a head injury because he was fighting them and was very uncooperative. We would call this the "fall in the hall" for the rest of our days. It was a pivotal moment in Bill's health.

When I got to the emergency room at about two o'clock in the morning, the doctor was evaluating him. He had not broken his nose or his knee, but he was quite bruised and still bleeding from the cut on his nose. He began to vomit, which is sometimes the sign of a brain injury, so he was admitted. I went home about 5:00 a.m. to rest and feed the dog. I returned about 10:00 a.m. He had two black eyes and a horribly bruised knee, but so far, all of his tests did not show he had injured his brain. He would probably need to stay in the hospital for a few days. I stayed all day and went home again for the night.

About three o'clock in the morning, the nurse called me and said, "Bill is very confused, pulling out his IV and very restless. We can't control him, can you come?" I said, "Of course, I'll be right there." Before I could leave the house, Bill called, "They have a scam going here, they are trying to tattoo me." He was obviously in trouble. I told him to put the nurse on the phone. "What's going on, why does he think you are going to tattoo him?" She answered, "We are just trying to restart his IV and he won't let us near him." I told the nurse I would be there as soon as I could - about 30 minutes.

When I got there, he was quiet again, but he would not let the nurses do anything for him. I helped them by giving him his pills and trying to calm him down. They got his IV restarted, and the doctor ordered a sedative for him, but he calmed down enough after I arrived that he didn't need to have it. I spent three days in the hospital with him. I never left except to get something to eat in the cafeteria. They had a chair for me to sleep in, but when he got confused after it got dark, I would get in bed with him to calm him down.

His mental confusion wasn't clearing up, especially at night, and I demanded another CT scan. I can get darn right "in your face, pushy" if I think Bill isn't getting the right care. I talked to the charge nurse and sort of "forced" her to call the doctor to get the scan. I wanted to be sure he was not bleeding in his brain, even though a CT scan had been done in the emergency room, and it didn't show anything.

Bill was taken to the x-ray department, and the scan was performed and fortunately, there was no problem with bleeding in his brain. The doctors decided he was probably coming down off all the drugs he had been taking for pain, and combined with the effects of the fall, it was hard for him to think clearly.

Because of his continued confusion at night, the doctor would not let him come home. He also needed some physical therapy for his knee. It was December 17th, and he was going to have to go to a skilled nursing facility for a few days. There were two available - one fairly close, the other further away. By the time the decision was made, he ended up in the one in Sacramento, the furthest away.

They wanted to have an ambulance take him, which I thought was unnecessary, so the nurses and I got him out to our car, then in the car, and I drove him to the facility. It was about four o'clock in the afternoon by the time we got him ready to go and in the car. The traffic was terrible, as it normally is at rush hour, but worse because Christmas was a week away.

Since there was still some daylight, his nighttime confusion had not set in. He was able to give me the directions to get to the facility since I wasn't familiar with the area. I was so happy to see that maybe getting him out of the hospital was making Bill feel better and clearing up his confusion. Bill was checked in and given some dinner, and I went home exhausted.

About two o'clock in the morning, I got a phone call from the nurse saying, "Bill would like some Tylenol." I thought, "Well just give it to him then." I didn't say that, but asked "Why are you calling me? Do you have to call the doctor?" They had called the doctor and got the order, but they were required to call the responsible party and let them know what was going on before giving the medication. I said, "Of course, give it to him as long as it is just plain Tylenol." I asked, "Why does he want it?" She told me, "He's not sleeping and has a headache."

The next day when I went to visit, he was in a different room. I asked, "What happened?" He told me, "After I got my Tylenol, my old roommate had a problem, so they moved me to a quieter room." His bed was by the door and he liked this room better as he could watch the people go by in the hall and see the TV better. His new roommate spent most of his time in the recreation room, so he had the room to himself most of the time.

I gave him his beloved newspapers, he ate breakfast and seemed to be resting quietly. He had not had any confusion during the night, thankfully. I talked to the dietitian about his food because he was very unhappy with what they were serving him. They said they would adjust the menu to his liking, and I was given permission to bring him food from the outside, like his favorite breakfast from McDonald's. Bill seemed happy in his new surroundings and was doing well, but I was not able to stay with him all day as I had when he was in the hospital. Being apart was hard for both of us.

He began physical therapy for his injured knee to make sure he could walk when he was discharged. They were also trying to build strength in his arms since he had been in bed recovering from surgery for so long before the fall. His incisions were not healing as well as they should have been, so the wound care nurse changed the dressing every day and made sure there was no infection. In general, he was doing fine, but the huge fall creating the "shake and rattle" to his head was going to take more time to heal.

When I went to visit him on December 24th, the nursing director asked me to come to her office to fill out some forms. He was only supposed to have been in the care facility a few days, and he had already been there almost a week. She told me, "Sometimes discharge is slower because therapy isn't going as well as expected and his wounds are not healing well."

She then told me that when he was admitted there had not been a mortuary listed on his admission papers. I just lost it, broke down in tears, and said, "No, that isn't necessary, he will be fine." It was Christmas, and she was talking about mortuaries, and I fell apart. I had held it together quite well until then. I told her to list the closest one since I didn't know of any. I had no idea where it was.

On Christmas day, I went to visit him and stayed for as long as they allowed me. I spent the rest of the day at home with the dog. He spent the rest of the day with all the other residents at the facility. We talked on the phone, and neither of us said it, but I knew we were both very lonely and feeling a little sad for ourselves. We decided not to open any presents until he returned home.

Bill was set to come home the next week, but as it turned out, he would be there six weeks. I caught a very bad cold and cough during that time and could not visit him. We talked on the phone, and he seemed to be in good spirits, but I know it was hard for him. The positive outcome of this was I discovered I could do quite well on my own while he was at rehab.

This was Bill's longest stay in a hospital. He was healing,

and his brain was coming back to its usual brilliant light. He was tired but still in recovery mode. I was worried about bringing him home, but I knew it was time. He certainly had enough hospital and rehab for a while.

Bill's walk was becoming more like a shuffle after the knee injury, combined with the previously broken ankle, but he was able to get around the house without a problem. He began to drive again because driving was important to Bill. He loved to get in the car and "go" to the grocery store, the library, and the lodge where we lived. Getting his freedom back was very healing for him. I started to relax a little, but not completely.

It was several months before Bill was back to the "old Bill" once again. He worked on his recovery every day, eating well, walking, and getting stronger. He returned to his customary routines eventually, and we were well on the way to leaving the "fall in the hall" to history.

Hypervigilance

Lesson: Emotional Freedom Tapping

Hypervigilance is the state or quality of being extremely alert or watchful. This is because when you're hypervigilant, your body stays in the state of "fight, flight, or freeze" that kicks in when you perceive a threat, whether it's real or not. Hypervigilance can cause extreme fatigue if one is in that mode for days, weeks, or months. The neurotransmitters that are responding in your body are in overdrive, and it's exhausting to the entire body. If this state doesn't cause extreme fatigue, it can cause insomnia. In my case, it was insomnia, I had always had trouble sleeping, but now it was much worse.

Loving and caring for Bill exacerbated my hypervigilance as I was so afraid of losing him. I believe hypervigilance happens naturally when someone is in a situation where poor health puts a loved one at risk. It is part of a relationship - being alert and always concerned about the other's welfare. I would never regret a minute of it, even though it was a difficult way to live.

I was hypervigilant before Bill fell, but it became even worse after the "fall in the hall." It was causing anxiety, and my adrenaline always seemed to be going at full speed. Most of the time, I kept things running smoothly and the house in order. Bill was taking his medication and eating well. We could still go out for coffee or lunch in a restaurant occasionally. Our "new normal" was developing as we created new ways of getting things done, like who took out the garbage and did the shopping. I tried to be around more but not make it seem like I was on guard all the time.

I was always in alert mode when he was up at night getting his glass of milk or a snack since that is when the fall took place. In general, he did not want help, and I was usually half asleep anyway, but I had a second sense as to what was going on in the kitchen. I may have looked asleep, but I was listening. Sometimes he would turn on the TV and watch the late news while he snacked and then come back to bed. I would finally settle to a sound sleep when I knew he was safely tucked back in bed. That is if I went back to sleep at all.

After he recovered, I was not really concerned about leaving him alone, even when I was gone all day. He would always promise to stay home even though he was able to drive a little. I had to trust him, or I would make myself crazy with worry. The fear of losing him or having him hurt someone else in a car accident was always on my mind when he drove by himself.

When Bill was strong enough to drive, he tended to be a fast driver, and that made me more concerned. He did not like me to comment on this, so I had to try and sit still and be quiet. I was taught to relieve some of the anxiety going on in my head by gently tapping my fingers on my other hand, side of my face, or arm to distract myself. Somewhere that he couldn't see.

This is called EFT or Emotional Freedom Tapping. It is used for anxiety, depression, headaches, pain, weight loss, and more. The main EFT tapping points are the side of the hand, eyebrow, the side of and under the eye, under the nose, chin, underarm, and top of the head. It's a simple technique, and I found it quite useful when my thoughts were running rampant in my head in what I called "anticipation" mode when I was thinking of what might happen next.

When I worked at the hospital, I would often try to avoid problems with a patient by anticipating what could happen. I basically predicted the future and acted upon it before it happened, like a drop in blood pressure or a heart arrhythmia. This saved many patients in the ICU where I worked, but it is mentally and physically exhausting.

This is what I started to do with Bill. If I could basically be a "fortune teller" and think ahead to what might happen, perhaps I could avoid a problem for him. I was right most of the time, but sometimes I did a lot of agonizing over something that never happened. The good thing is, I was prepared if he were to have another medical issue. The problem with this is that I couldn't see inside his body to see what might happen next.

Depression is common among caregivers, as well as other emotional problems. Sleep deprivation also wreaks havoc on an already tired body. Always listening for sounds of a fall or a cough, or the shouting of, "I need help," is mentally and physically draining. This all leads to caregiver burnout. Signs of burnout include lack of interest in previously enjoyed activities, difficulty sleeping, socially withdrawing, irritability, feelings of sadness, unhealthy eating, and more alcohol use.

I had to look deep into myself to find ways to avoid "burnout." But what began to happen, and this is frequent with caregivers, is I began to ignore some of my own health issues. It was easy to tell myself that I wasn't sick or didn't feel bad until it happened so often, and with such intensity, it could not be ignored. I began to develop health problems that could lead to my inability to care for Bill.

Our answer for my "burnout and stress" became our beloved dog, Grace. She managed my hypervigilance by getting me to walk her every day, forcing me to enjoy the outdoors and appreciate the thirty minutes of quiet. She woke me early to feed her, and we enjoyed the quiet while we watched the sunrise admiring the start of another day.

Grace was my dog, but she adored Bill. I would tell her, "Go find Dad." She would scamper off to find Bill in his chair or in bed. If he were in bed, he would drop his hand down and pet her, so she knew he was there. When he got up, she would greet him in the hallway, and they would sit on the couch by the windows of the kitchen so they could watch the world go by. She barked at people walking by, the UPS man, the mail lady, and anyone else she felt she needed to "talk" to.

Grace had many friends in the neighborhood she visited when I walked her in the mornings. She kept me company when Bill slept and was always my shadow. She would panic if she couldn't find me. You cannot help but smile when a dog is in your life and loves you no matter what your health problems are. Grace was a wonderful companion to us while Bill was not feeling well. A sure sign he wasn't feeling great on any given day was if he raised his voice and yelled,

"Grace, quit barking!" as loud as possible.

Studies have shown that interacting with animals helps lower blood pressure, reduce anxiety, and decrease depression. This can increase levels of the hormone oxytocin, which can slow a person's heart rate and breathing, lower blood pressure, and inhibit the production of stress hormones. All these changes help create a sense of calm and comfort.

Pets don't judge or try to give advice or ask questions. They don't need reassurance that everything will be okay. They live day by day and are there when you need them to show affection, be a companion, and offer comfort (Source: Cancer.net).

These earlier days of caregiving were just the beginning of what I would need to do for Bill. We soon forgot his long stay in the hospital and began to live our quiet life again. I would always be worried about another fall or that another surgery would be needed, but I was beginning to feel a little more relaxed that he was okay. Grace, of course, was always at our side, doing her part to keep us happy and calm

Cardioversion One

Lesson: Whether a good decision or not, it's Bill's decision

Bill's long hospital stay was soon forgotten, and he was back to being himself again. Driving, grocery shopping, cooking, and visiting with friends at the lodge. Life was good. The holidays were approaching, and they always made us smile with all the decorations, lights, and good food.

A couple of weeks before Christmas, we attended a luncheon for Bill's History Group that he attended meetings for once a month. He loved the group, and I knew some of the people who were part of the group, so I went as well. We finished lunch, and as we were leaving, Bill looked at me and said, "We better go home; I don't feel well." We drove home, and he went to bed and took a long nap. He looked okay, just tired, and so I didn't think much about it.

He got up later in the afternoon, we had a small dinner and were watching TV. He looked up at me again and said, "I don't feel good, I don't feel right." I went over to him, helped him up, and walked him to the bedroom so he could lay down again. I held his hand while we walked down the hall, and I thought his skin felt a bit clammy, and his color wasn't good at all. I said to him, "Lay down for a bit and I'll take your blood pressure, but I need to find my stethoscope."

I went to find my stethoscope, and when I returned, his color was ashen. I took his pulse and blood pressure, which was low, and listened to his heart. I said, "Bill you are in atrial fib, we have to get you to the emergency room." He asked, "What's atrial fib?"

I gave him the brief definition. "Your heart is beating at an irregular rate and the blood does not circulate into your body. It can cause blood clots and possibly a stroke. It's very dangerous and needs to be taken care of immediately." He said, "Okay, get me to the hospital." I got him in the car and drove the half-hour to the hospital to get him to the emergency room.

A more accurate medical definition of atrial fibrillation is an irregular and often rapid heart rate that occurs when the two upper chambers of the heart experience chaotic electrical signals. The result is a fast and irregular heart rhythm. The heart rate in atrial fibrillation may range from about 30 to 175 beats a minute. If a patient is attached to a cardiac monitor, the wave of the line designating the heart rate is very irregular without the normal configuration you would see for a normal heart rhythm – called sinus rhythm. It can speed up, slow down and have long pauses before the next heartbeat.

Atrial fibrillation is one of the more common causes of stroke in the elderly. The two upper chambers of the heart, called the atrium, are beating chaotically, while the lower chambers of the heart, the ventricles, are not. The blood can sit in the ventricles rather than circulating, where it pools and begins to clot. When the heart then has a normal heartbeat that involves the ventricles, the blood is pushed out to circulate, and the blood clots can then travel to the rest of the body, most likely the head. This causes a stroke by blocking off one of the blood vessels in the brain. It can go to other areas of the body as well, but the ramifications of a blood clot in the brain are very serious and life-threatening.

Bill was immediately put on a cardiac monitor, and an IV was started to give a drug that could stop the irregular heart rate. The nurses knew that I was a nurse and could read the monitor and "read" what his heart was doing. I also knew when Bill had a grey pallor, that they might not notice because they were in and out of the room so quickly, that he was in trouble. After several hours his heart rate did not return to normal, and it was determined at about 2:00 a.m. that he needed to be "cardioverted."

The medical definition of cardioversion is to send an electric shock to the heart through electrodes placed on the chest. This is indeed a medical emergency, and several doctors and nurses are present when it is performed. If you have ever watched a medical show on TV, the scene might go much like this:

The patient may or may not be sedated, depending on how quickly the procedure must be done. The defibrillator used for cardioversion has two "paddles" that are lubricated with a clear gel. This keeps the skin from burning when they are held against the body to administer the electoral charge.

Someone is holding the paddles on the patient's chest, one in about the center, the other on the side; someone yells "charge," and the amount of electrical charge required is set on the machine. Then the one holding the paddles yells, "clear," which means everyone needs to get away from the bed because if you are touching it, you could get shocked too. A button on each paddle is pushed simultaneously to send the charge through the patient's heart and hopefully reset the chaotic signal that is causing the irregular heartbeat.

The patient sort of lifts off the bed as the electricity goes through the body. The heart is set back to a normal rhythm if all goes well. It just takes a few seconds. Sometimes this is repeated if the heart does not respond with the first jolt of electricity. The amount of electricity is increased, and the shock is given again. The amount of electricity given can be from 50 to 300 joules. It is very dramatic, and every nurse I ever knew, including myself, shivered with anxiety the first time they cardioverted a patient.

When they were about to cardiovert Bill, the nurses asked me to leave, well, actually they told me to leave. I told them I would go outside the door, but I would not leave as I knew exactly what they were doing.

As I stood outside the door, they sedated him, and the cardioversion was done. Bill's heart responded immediately, converting to a normal heartbeat with only one shock. But then Bill would not wake up from the sedation. Several people yelled at him, "Mr. Attwater, wake up, it's all over, you're fine." This was repeated several times.

They should have just called him "Bill," it was such a formal salutation that I don't think he even registered they were calling his name. He always said Mr. Attwater was his dad, not him. After several minutes, he still wouldn't wake up. I walked in, pushed my way through the crowd to the head of the bed and grabbed his arms, leaned into his ear, and said, "Bill, wake up, you are all right. It's all over, please don't make me call your kids." He started to come around. The nurses laughed and said, "We will have to remember that threat for the future."

Bill woke up and responded appropriately after the sedation and cardioversion, but we did not get to go home right away as he thought we would. They had to keep him on the heart monitor for a while and make sure he could stand, walk and go to the bathroom. Then all the medications we would take home started to roll in. Lots of them!

He was given a pill, known as a beta-blocker, to stop the atrial fib from happening, and an anticoagulant, first in the form of a shot and then in a pill. Since the risk of a blood clot is high with atrial fib and there was a good chance he would have it again, he would have to take an anticoagulant for the rest of his life.

Bill would first be given shots of Heparin to keep his blood from clotting and then eventually would go on an oral medication called Coumadin, also known as Warfarin, commonly called a "blood thinner." The pills available now for anticoagulation that have far fewer rules and side effects were not available at this time.

The shots were easy for me to give at home, but they are odd in that they are given in the abdomen. Bill would cringe when he saw the needle as it is a bit painful to have a shot in the tummy, even if you have some fat there. Coumadin, on the other hand, is a very difficult pill to take with lots of dietary limitations, and frequent blood draws. Bill quickly learned to hate this pill because of these rules.

Fortunately, we lived near the lab, but the blood needed to be drawn first thing in the morning, so he would get up and get to the lab very early, hopefully before the crowds. The blood test is the International Normalized Ratio (INR) that determines how anticoagulated someone's blood is. A result of 1.0 up to 1.5 is normal. A lower INR result means your blood is "not thin enough" or coagulates too quickly and puts you at risk of developing a blood clot. A high INR means your blood coagulates too slowly, and you are at risk of bleeding.

Since the pill is an anticoagulant, you can't eat anything that is a natural coagulant. The biggest thing being lettuce and green leafy vegetables because they have vitamin K in them that cause blood to clot. In fact, a vitamin K shot is the antidote to Coumadin if too much is taken. Alcohol causes problems, as well, by keeping the blood from clotting while taking Coumadin.

By the afternoon after the blood draw, someone from the Coumadin Clinic would call and tell him what medication adjustments to make based on the results. He could be adding, or subtracting pills, including cutting them in half. It's an agonizing process to get the drug regulated, and if you just happen to have eaten something with vitamin K in it the day before, the test can be thrown off easily. At one time, Bill's INR was 6.5. That is extremely high, and the clinic said to skip a few days of pills. I suggested, "Don't fall on your head or work with knives in the kitchen. You'll bleed to death if you cut yourself." I was trying to be funny; he didn't see it that way.

All the rules of what to eat and the frequent blood draws were just too much for Bill. He wasn't feeling quite back to normal yet with the new heart medications, so he decided that he would stop taking the coumadin. I was overwrought with worry about this decision, but as it was his to make, I had to stay quiet and let him make his own decision.

He continued without the Coumadin for several months without an issue. He felt better and ate what he wanted without restrictions. Once again, we were back to life as normal at our house, and life moved on. It always seemed there was something lurking in the background that would change this that we had no control over. I just prayed it didn't happen too soon.

Chemical Cardioversion

Lesson: Breathe Bill – a Few Minutes of Deep Breathing Can Reduce Stress

Just when we thought we were doing fine and all was well, atrial fib struck Bill for the second time. One evening he looked at me and said once again, "I don't feel good." I checked his pulse, and he was in atrial fib with a rate between 90 to 110 beats per minute.

Off we go to the emergency room again for another night of sedation, cardioversion, and long waits. I was not calling an ambulance for him at this time because although he felt bad, he was not in any distress. He was breathing normally, his color was okay, and so I was comfortable driving him.

Of course, every time you go to the emergency room, you have a different doctor. This doctor did not want to cardiovert with electricity as we had before but wanted to try the same IV medication Bill had the first time that would hopefully stop the heart's chaotic rhythm. Bill's cardiologist had told me he didn't want the medication used again because it didn't work the first time. The ER doctor would not listen to me. It would take a few hours, but it was worth the try in his mind. This is called chemical cardioversion.

The IV was started, and the medication was set to drip in via an IV infusion pump. Any medication like this that can have potent effects on the heart is given with an infusion pump so the speed of the infusion can be controlled. Sometimes IVs can be what is called "positional," and if the arm is moved, the rate the fluid goes in speeds up, slows down, or can stop. This could be dangerous with this drug as if it did not go in at a set rate, it might not do its job - that is, stopping the atrial fib.

Bill began to fall asleep as we were approaching midnight. He has sleep apnea, and when he sleeps without his CPAP machine, he can stop breathing or snore. This happened several times, and when the monitor would alarm because it did not detect breathing, I would yell at him, "Breathe, Bill." About halfway through the infusion, the alarm was slightly different sounding, and I looked up at the monitor. There was a flat line - Bill's heart had stopped.

I jumped up to help him, and the nurses came running in at the same time. I backed away as they began their work. One nurse started CPR and others got the equipment ready to shock his heart to a normal rhythm. This is like cardioversion, but this time it was to restart his heart. After what seemed like forever, but according to the monitor was a very short time, his heart restarted again without the shock being given. Everyone then relaxed. Well, the nurses did. I'm not sure I ever did. It seems the flat line, or no pulse, was the pause his heart took to restart a normal rhythm.

The cardiologist told me later that not using the CPAP machine can cause atrial fib, heart disease, and stroke. Using the CPAP machine improves the sleep cycle and can prevent daytime fatigue. Bill was a good patient, though, and always used the machine when he slept or took a nap at home. So, I'm not sure that his problems were related to being without the machine in the ER. You can't wear it all day, every day, only when sleeping, so it had to be a heart issue, not a CPAP issue. CPAP stands for Continuous Positive Airway Pressure. By sending a positive pressure of air into the airway, it prevents snoring and maintains a constant flow of air into the lungs.

We were eventually sent home with more drugs to try to keep the atrial fib at bay, but mostly a new anticoagulant, this time a new pill that did not require the dietary restrictions and lab work to determine the dose. The only issue with this pill is that there is no antidote if one were to take too much or had a severe injury with a lot of bleeding. As I write this, I understand there is an antidote that can be used now, but at that time, there was none. This pill, called Pradaxa, is taken twice a day and didn't have any known side effects, like many of the other heart medications that Bill was taking.

Bill was seen by another cardiologist after this happened and given a thorough battery of tests for his heart. He was still having atrial fib occasionally, so more beta-blockers were added to his list of pills. Their job is to prevent atrial fib, but they also cause drowsiness as it seems they slow everything down, not just the heart. They make the heart beat more slowly and with less force which also lowers the blood pressure so that they can prevent high blood pressure as well.

Once again, we settled into the new pill regimen, and

Bill was feeling pretty good. Until one summer day that was painfully hot –105 degrees, Bill had atrial fib again. He disappeared into the bedroom, I thought for a nap, but a few minutes later, he came out to the living room to find me. "My pulse is 38!" I jumped up, made him sit down, and checked his pulse again. Yes, it was that low. He was feeling a little dizzy, but not too bad, he reported. This time I called an ambulance.

They arrived quickly and put him on the monitor that showed he was in a very slow atrial fib, less than 40 beats per minute. They started an IV and gave him a huge amount of fluids because of the heat outside. They wanted to be sure he was not dehydrated. They finally loaded him in the ambulance, and off they went. I followed later with the CPAP machine, just in case he had to stay.

When I arrived, Bill still had a very slow heart rate. The doctor came in to see him and said he was "overly beta-blocked." Beta-blockers are the medications that make the heart beat more slowly and with less force, which lowers blood pressure. They are also used to stop atrial fibrillation. Bill was on a very high dose of two of these drugs. The medication he was taking for his high blood pressure combined with the medication for the atrial fib had dropped his pulse too low.

The doctor admitted him to make sure his heart rate didn't get any lower. I stayed with him for quite a while, and he was giving me a list of the things he wanted me to bring him for his hospital stay. The same doctor walked in a few hours later and said, "I'm sending you home. You'll be fine, lots of people walk around with a pulse of 38." I stood up and said, "Are you kidding, the people with a pulse of 38 are athletes, Bill can hardly walk." We were sent home with the directions to go back to the ER if he had any problems. They always tell you that, like it's the easiest thing in the world to get there.

I thought it was a terrible decision, but the doctor would not change her mind. We were to see a cardiologist later in the week and prayed that nothing happened before that appointment. My hypervigilance kicked in, and I watched Bill closely and checked his pulse so frequently that he would "shoo" me away. I knew he was worried too, but there wasn't much else we could do but worry.

As it turned out, the rest of the week went by without incident. We were to go to the cardiologist on a Friday, which is the day they put in pacemakers at this facility, but no one told us this. If we had known, they would have put one in that day. Once it was decided Bill would need a pacemaker, an appointment was made for the next Friday. He would have to wait another very long week before it was put in and then he could start taking more beta-blockers to stop the atrial fib.

I wondered, what happens when the spouse or loved one does not know how to check a pulse for an abnormal heartbeat or take blood pressure? My guess is they worry less because they don't know what is going on. I had to quit "thinking" and just move on with the week. It would do no good, and I would have enough to worry about when they put the pacemaker in.

Pacemaker

Lesson: Bill Knows What is Best for Bill

Our visit to the cardiologist was an easy trip. Bill could walk a longer distance while using his walker, and I didn't have to push him in a wheelchair from the parking lot. The doctor was very friendly and thorough, and after a long talk, it was decided that Bill would get a pacemaker.

The beta-blockers keeping his heart out of atrial fib had to be increased, and this could not be done without the pacemaker as a backup to keep his heart beating above sixty beats per minute. They are easy to live with, and Bill wouldn't even know he had it after the incision healed. What I was concerned about was Bill having another surgery.

The following Friday, a week away, he was admitted to have the procedure done. It was performed in a normal surgery suite because all the equipment is there with the necessary personnel to handle an emergency, if one occurs, while the pacemaker is being inserted. It was getting late in the afternoon; we had waited a long time, and they had not taken him into surgery yet. He was getting restless and very uncomfortable.

The doctor came out to the waiting area, "I apologize for being late and keeping you waiting." He explained the surgery would start soon. Bill was exhausted, not doing great laying on the uncomfortable gurney, but to be frank, I thought the doctor looked worse. It was his fourth pacemaker insertion of the day. I wanted to tell him we would come back after he took a nap.

Pacemaker insertions are generally quick and easy. The cardiologist makes about a 2-inch cut just below the collarbone, usually on the left side of the chest, and inserts the pacemaker's wires into a vein. These wires, called pacing leads, are guided along the vein into the correct chambers of the heart, where they are then lodged into the tissue of the heart. The wires are guided by the doctor as he watches on an x-ray to be sure he does not pierce the heart or a blood vessel with them. If that happened, it would require open-heart surgery to repair it, which is another reason why the pacemaker is put in while the patient is in a surgical suite.

Once the leads are settled into the heart, the opposite ends are connected to the pacemaker. Then it is fitted into a small pocket created between the skin of the upper chest and the chest muscle. The incision is closed with surgical tape, and the patient then wears a sling on the arm on the side where the pacemaker was inserted. This is so the wires can implant themselves in the heart without being dislodged by movement. Bill was not told he would have to do this before the surgery and was not happy about it. He quit wearing it after about ten days.

The doctor told me the pacemaker insertion went well, but Bill started to cough partway through the procedure, and they could not keep him lying flat as they needed to for the surgery. He was given several breathing treatments, and finally, they were able to proceed. I was not surprised; Bill often has breathing issues while under anesthesia. He is a big guy and does not tolerate lying flat very well, which can compromise his breathing. He was admitted for the night because it was so late in the day and so his breathing could be monitored. They didn't want to send him home in case he had more breathing problems. He would have several more breathing treatments during the night.

After he was settled, I went home for the night and returned the next day to find him in an uproar. He had been placed in an overflow area of the recovery room where it was noisy, and there was always someone bustling about. The patient next to him kept screaming, "Get me out of this hell hole." I had to agree, and Bill was with him completely, but he was the biggest source of the noise. I felt so sorry for Bill because he had no sleep and just wanted to go home.

Eventually, he was discharged, and I drove him home. Our friend Chris came to help me get him out of the car since Bill could not use his left arm to push his way out of the car seat. We got him into bed and settled, and his friend then left. "Call me if you need me, I'm only ten minutes away." He said this every time he left the house.

Bill slept for most of the day, but now the fun began as I had to nag him to wear the sling so he did not move his left arm away from his body. He can be very stubborn and was not interested in following this rule. I begged him to leave the sling on and told him, "If you dislodge the leads, you will have to go through the whole surgery again." It didn't matter. He knew he would be okay. "I'll be fine, just let me sleep."

A month later, we went to the cardiologist for a "pacemaker check." They can determine how much the pacemaker has been used or "pacing" by connecting it to a computer with a strange apparatus they placed around Bill's neck. It would also check to see if he was still having atrial fib. Pacemakers don't stop atrial fib; instead, it would override Bill's slow heartbeat caused by the beta-blockers. This is called a "demand pacemaker," so if his pulse dropped below 60, the pacemaker would kick in and keep his pulse at 60 or above.

The tech then told us that Bill had dislodged one of the leads, but since it was attached to the chamber of his heart that he did not need "paced," it would probably be okay. I wanted to walk over and knock Bill on the head. I generally don't say anything in front of medical staff unless it is a gentle suggestion, but I couldn't help myself. "I told you that you needed to keep that sling on." He just smiled and didn't say a word.

We were told, "I'm sure the pacemaker will be fine, and you won't have to go back to surgery, but you need to be careful for a while." I was still beside myself with exasperation as this was so easily prevented. We got home, and not another word was said about it, despite my wanting to say, "I told you so!" It would do no good at this point, so I just left it alone. I waited for the call to tell us he needed to go back to surgery. Thankfully, it never came.

This was when I began to realize that no matter how much I loved and took care of Bill, it was his decision as to what happened to his body. It was hard sometimes to watch this happen when I thought I knew better. But it was his life, therefore his decisions. My medical background would often conflict with some of his ideas, but I had to be true to him.

The medical profession now emphasizes that patients play a key role in managing their health and should always be actively supported when making decisions. They accept the patient as "the expert" when it comes to their own care, when appropriate. The patient must be mentally fit and well enough to make decisions. If they are not, then the family must get involved in the process. The patient's values and preferences must be regarded by the health care team whenever a care plan is made or a need for a procedure is made. I would have to do the same.

After Bill's surgery, we were given a device about the size of a phone to hold over the pacemaker to do "pacemaker checks," through an app on my cell phone. Once every three months, I would hold it over the pacemaker and hit the "go" button, and over a few minutes, it would send a report to the pacemaker clinic through the phone. The information included how often the pacemaker was used and how much atrial fib Bill was having. We would never hear back, which I thought was curious, but then again, "no news was good news" in this case. I did this check every three months, and we went into the clinic once a year, until the pandemic struck, and then we no longer visited the clinic.

The pacemaker insertion site soon healed, and the scar disappeared. It was like he had never had anything done. The good news now being that his heart rate would never drop below sixty, and perhaps all the beta-blockers he was taking were doing their job to prevent atrial fib and eliminate the potential for a stroke.

Kidney Stones

Lesson: Take Control of Your Diet

Bill had been plagued with kidney stones for most of his life. Over twenty stones over a span of forty years or so. Painful, drop you to your knees, gut-wrenching pain caused by tiny stones that get caught in the ureter between the kidney and the bladder. Before I knew him, he had been in the hospital several times for a day or two to manage the pain with narcotic pain medication. For a man, it is the closest thing to childbirth they will ever experience. It's that painful to pass a kidney stone!

Bill woke up one morning with the horrible pain and the feeling of doom of another kidney stone. We went to the emergency room for the usual pain medication and CT scan to see where it was located. This stone was different; it was too high to pass on its own and way too big. Bill tried for days to pass the stone; it would not move. He wasn't in a lot of pain at this time, but that worried us more as we were wondering if he would ever pass it. He would know if it moved as the pain would increase.

We then had an appointment with a urologist who told Bill he had a few options. The wait and see option that he was not eager to do. Lithotripsy, which is a medical procedure that uses shock waves or a laser to break down stones in the kidney or ureter. The remaining small particles of stone would then come out when he urinated. Or he could have a surgery called ureteroscopy.

During ureteroscopy, the surgeon inserts a narrow, flexible instrument called a ureteroscope through the urethral opening, passing it through the bladder to where the stone is in the ureter or kidney. A small laser located at the end of the ureteroscope would break up and remove the stone. Bill chose this surgery as he thought it would get the stone out faster and easier.

This surgery was performed as an outpatient procedure with general anesthesia, which at this point, Bill was tolerating fairly well. He had all the labs and checks done by a pre-surgery doctor that said he was healthy enough for the surgery. I agreed but worried as I knew how Bill's lungs often reacted poorly to the tube in his throat for the ventilator used during surgery.

The day of surgery was moving along well until it was his time to go into the operating room. An emergency surgery had bumped Bill out of line. He waited patiently but was a little frustrated. The doctor came to talk to him and assured him, "You'll be next, it won't be long."

He then told Bill, "You'll leave here with a small tube in your bladder that will extend about 24 inches. This will allow the stone fragments to pass without difficulty." Glancing at me he says, "Your wife can pull it out in a week." No one asked me if this was okay. I was just told to do it. Bill did not seem pleased with this because he thought once the surgery was done, he would be through with the stone forever.

The surgery went well, Bill had a little difficulty with breathing, but they took care of that with a breathing treatment in the recovery room. He stayed for a few hours, and I brought him home. Bill slept for days, as he always does to recover. The only problem was he constantly felt like he had to "pee" because of the tube that was in place. His urine was blood-tinged as well, but we were warned about this.

I woke Bill frequently and made him drink water to keep the urine flowing and the stone fragments moving through the system. He didn't mind this, and with his usual good nature, drank the water and went back to sleep or urinated and then went back to sleep. If I didn't wake him up, he would have slept all night, and urine would not have been as free-flowing to remove the stone fragments.

While he was resting, I began to probe the internet for more information about how to stop kidney stones. Bill had always talked about eliminating spinach and Swiss chard, but I wondered if there was more he could do to prevent more stones from forming.

I found there is a recommended diet one should follow when you have kidney stones. Bill was pretty good at following some of the diet, by mostly eliminating the foods he didn't like, but it was difficult for him to follow all the recomendations. He was still doing the cooking at this time, so I didn't have much control over what he ate.

A plant-based diet is thought to be ideal, except there are some vegetables high in oxalates that form the kidney stones. Chocolate, beets, nuts, tea, rhubarb, spinach, Swiss chard, and sweet potatoes are high in oxalates. Bill eliminated spinach and Swiss chard and thought that was all he needed to do.

Many sources of protein, such as red meat, pork, chicken, poultry, fish, and eggs, increase the amount of uric acid produced, which can also cause gout. Eating large amounts of protein also reduces a chemical in urine called citrate, which prevents the formation of kidney stones.

Alternatives to animal protein include quinoa, tofu (bean curd), hummus, chia seeds, and Greek yogurt. These alternatives made us laugh out loud. There was no way Bill was going to replace meat with tofu.

The recommendation to prevent kidney stones involves several things:

- Drink at least twelve 8-ounce glasses of water daily
- Drink citrus juices, such as orange juice
- Eat a calcium-rich food at each meal, at least three times daily
- Limit your intake of animal protein
- Eat less salt, added sugar, and products containing high fructose corn syrup
- Avoid foods and drinks high in oxalates and phosphates
- Avoid eating or drinking anything that dehydrates you, such as alcohol

I found all of this very interesting in that the doctor never gave any of these recommendations to us. It seems that dietary changes never get mentioned by doctors. There is a philosophy that if you go to a surgeon, you are going to have surgery. That's what they do. They are not dietitians, so if you want dietary information, you need to go elsewhere, like a dietitian.

Bill rested and recovered from the anesthesia after a few days and seemed to pass the stone fragments without difficulty. I pulled the little tube out that had been left in after surgery, and all seemed to be fine. I showed him what I had found about diet, and he agreed it was sound advice. As I suspected, almost all the recommendations would be ignored, except he had always been a good water drinker, so he would continue to follow that recommendation.

A few years later, we would find out changing his diet to a plant-based diet could have possibly slowed his decline and prevented some other medical issues like cognitive decline. Again, we were looking to the future and trying to guess what would happen, but Bill would show no interest in changing his diet. It caused nothing but a battle, and as he says, "I'm 83, I must have done something right to live so long."

Fortunately, it seemed to be the end of his kidney stones, but he can remember every stone he had and how much pain they gave him. It made for a great story when someone else said they've had a kidney stone. Bill would match them chapter and verse regarding pain, medication, and trips to the ER.

Our Final Trip

Lesson: Enjoy the Last Dance

In 2016, a few years before Bill became seriously ill, he received an invitation from his law school, the University of Washington, to attend the fiftieth anniversary of his graduating class. It was going to be in Seattle and would take a lot of maneuvering to make it happen, but I was determined we would go. Flights, rental cars, and a hotel that Bill could get in and out of with ease were the high priority, as his ankle was giving him a great deal of pain at this time.

Bill didn't really want to go, but I thought this was a great opportunity for him to see his old alma mater and Seattle one last time. "Come on Bill, this will be fun, and you may never have the chance to get up there again," He lamented. "I don't want to go, it's too much trouble." With a big smile on my face, I said, "I'll do everything, you just have to pick out an outfit. We even have mileage, so you won't have to pay for the flights." He gently nodded his consent. I was on the computer that very afternoon arranging everything. I talked this trip up like it was the biggest trip we would ever take. It wasn't, but it, unfortunately, would be the last trip for us.

Bill told me, "No one will remember me, I graduated seven months early and didn't attend the ceremony." I didn't think this was important as most of the class probably wouldn't be there anyway, and it didn't matter if anyone remembered anyone else. I was sure they would all have great stories to tell about their careers. Fifty years out from graduation is a long time, and it was possible many were not even still alive.

Bill's parents had lived in Seattle at one time as well, and he had fond memories of his time there with them. We also used to go into Seattle when we lived on Whidbey Island for eight years. It was a ferry ride and about a 90-minute drive into the center of Seattle from where we lived. I thought it would be fun for us to go back and visit with all these memories knowing we would have plenty to talk about while we were there.

We flew up a day early so we could wander around and visit one of our favorite restaurants while we were there. Our hotel was right on the water, we could walk across the street to the restaurant, and I could wander the downtown area while Bill napped. The afternoon before the party we decided to drive around and find the restaurant where the reunion was going to be held and do a little sightseeing. Bill was still driving, so I was glad I did not have to maneuver the traffic in Seattle.

Bill found his parent's old home just a short distance from where the party was going to take place. His memories of his mother and father living in this home are precious. He lived there too, for a while, and described the inside of the house and told me all about the neighbors that were there at the time and what was happening in everyone's life. Of course, everyone had moved on by then, but these memories were so sweet they almost made me tear up.

The party was to be held in a restaurant on the water where the cruise ships come in, a lovely setting for remembering old school days. We didn't know how many people were going to attend, but the restaurant was quite large, so it seemed everyone should fit in just fine. The view was spectacular as well, so we were anticipating a lovely evening.

We dressed early and drove to the restaurant to find parking close to the door for Bill. I wore pants and a sweater with a little jacket, and Bill wore slacks and a pullover sweater that made him look very dashing. We didn't think there was a serious dress code for this event, so we made our outfits easy to pack and travel with.

We entered the lovely restaurant and found the room where the party was being held. We had already chosen the food we would be eating when we returned the invitation and told the organizers we were coming. We got a drink and wandered the room a while, Bill talking to people he knew or thought he remembered while we were getting comfortable with the setting. As it turned out, there were only about fifteen graduates from his class, and some had their spouses with them for a total of about twenty-five people in the room.

We sat down to eat and visit with our table mates, and this was when the fun began. The organizer of the party asked every graduate to talk about their careers. I thought, oh no, this will go on forever, but these men, there were no female graduates there, had some great stories to tell. I was entranced as each person took his turn to talk.

The man sitting with his wife next to Bill had been a judge in Arizona, and the couple next to me were the heir and now owner, of a large jewelry store chain. He never worked as a lawyer but did interesting things in Japan before he took over the family jewelry store. Another of the men had defended someone that had been caught on the show, "America's Most Wanted." And then Bill spoke up and talked about his work and his two visits to the United States Supreme Court. He mentioned the day Clint Eastwood came to his office unannounced and got all the secretaries in a dither. He also spoke of the wonderful relationships he had with all the governors he worked with in California.

The final question asked by the organizer was, "Who traveled the furthest to come to the party?" It turned out to be us. We received a bottle of wine and some University of Washington memorabilia – two ball caps and two coffee mugs. We had to give the wine to one of our table mates because we couldn't travel home with it on the plane. It was such a fun and enjoyable evening, considering Bill had to be talked into going, he did enjoy himself.

We flew home the next day with wonderful memories of this trip. Little did we know at the time that it would be our last flight to anywhere. I was so happy I pushed Bill into going as he enjoyed it more than he expected. I enjoyed it too, and that's often not the case when I'm with people Bill knows or worked with and I don't know them.

A few days after we got home Bill received a certificate from the California State Bar congratulating him for being a member for fifty years. It's very impressive and a beautiful remembrance of his years as an attorney. Even after he retired, he was often asked to do depositions and answer questions for the people who worked in his old office. He loved his job and is very proud of his accomplishments. These two events made Bill smile for the rest of his life.

The certificate hangs over his desk along with the cards he was given when he went to the United States Supreme Court. It is truly a wall of accomplishments.

Walking Devices and Wheelchairs

Lesson: Gentle Convincing

Medical problems continued to mount up for Bill, and his walk was becoming more and more painful. He began to shuffle his feet rather than picking them up in a normal "step." His right ankle was beginning to "cave" in, and the ankle bone was becoming more and more prominent, sticking out in the wrong direction as he changed his gait to accommodate for the pain.

It was clear to me that another big fall was on the horizon if he didn't get some support while walking. I suggested a cane, but he just grimaced. "I don't want to look like an old man." I jokingly said, "But you are an old man." He didn't laugh, and I figured I would have to come up with a new approach to get him to use a cane.

We were out shopping for groceries one day and right across the street was the medical equipment store. I suggested we stop and just look at the canes and other mobility devices. He frowned, but he was always such a good sport at anything I suggested, we stopped.

The owner of the store knew Bill and was quite friendly with him. They always had long talks about absolutely everything when he had stopped in at other times. I thought she might help me to convince him a cane was a good idea. She asked if she could help us find anything, and I told her, "I think Bill needs a cane, maybe you could show us the best options for him." She agreed and began showing Bill all the different types. Who knew there were so many?

The handles varied quite a bit, from a curved handle with specific places to put your fingers and thumb, a straight one that was like a stick, also a curved handle, like a shepherd's crook, or a handle shaped like a "T," as well as those that had the head of an animal, like a lion that you grasped, or they could have a knob, like a doorknob.

The bottoms of the cane were also different as some were just the single tip that hit the floor with a rubber cover on it, or there were some that had three or four tips that touched the floor so the cane couldn't fall over. I joked, "It's like a tricycle for the beginning cane user." No one laughed. I decided just to let him try them all and see if he would purchase one.

I had a "cane" education that day. The "handle" or the part you would hold could be as varied as the colors and materials the canes were made of. This store carried metal canes primarily, with a plastic or rubber type handle, but wooden ones were available at other specialty stores. The "collar" is the band or ring that refers to the flange or ring where the handle joins to the shaft. The "shaft" is the straight part of the cane, which can be made from anything, it seems, that can be made long enough and strong enough to support a person's weight.

And here is the name I never knew and never would have guessed. The part of the cane that hits the floor is called the "ferrule." This is the rubber part of the cane, on the current ones, that shields the rest of the cane from puddles and mud or snow. Older canes did not have this, and they would deteriorate rapidly if exposed to the elements for very long. And finally, beneath the handle, there is often an "eyelet" where a fabric-type loop is placed that one can put over their wrist so they don't drop the cane.

Bill decided on a simple cane with a handle that had a rubber grip that extended out like a "gun." Plain blue and very easy to adjust to his height. He didn't like the little loop to put over his wrist so he wouldn't lose it, so the owner offered him this little device that you put on the cane called a crutch or cane holder.

You placed it up by the top of the cane, near the handle. It had about a quarter-sized rubber piece that stuck out that you could hang on a table or a counter. The rubber piece kept the cane from slipping off and falling to the floor. I think that's what sold him, as it was a nifty invention in his mind. He went through several of these over the years because they did fall off if you weren't careful.

The cane was taken home and left in the car. I was only going to fight one "battle" a day, so I left it there and didn't say a word. I would leave it to him to determine if it was the right time to use it. As always, this was his life and his decision to make.

Within a short time, Bill was beginning to have more trouble walking, so I brought the cane in and said, "Why don't you try this and see if it helps you?" He made a face, but he did try it and decided it did take the weight off his ankle, so he continued to use it.

Soon, one cane became five canes. If he saw one that was interesting looking, like a lion's head for a handle, he bought it, or I did. Canes made of several different colors and materials began to show up at the house. Eventually, there would be a cane located at every doorway of the house just in case he didn't grab one when he got out of his chair.

We also lost a few at the grocery store by leaving them in the cart after shopping and putting the groceries in the car. He would get home, determine he had forgotten it, and call the store. Some Good Samaritan had usually turned it in, and I would go pick it up. There were also times when he would go somewhere, lose the cane, and have no idea where he left it, and it would be lost forever.

Eventually, I could see that Bill could use more support when he walked. The cane was not enough, so I stopped at the medical supply store again and bought him a walker. It was a large enough walker that he could sit on it if he got tired. It, too, sat for a while before it was used, but I knew it would come in handy one day.

That day came soon for Bill. He just couldn't get down the hall without a lot of help. He was in too much pain and very weak. I put the walker in front of him and said, "Try this, I bet it will help!" He tried it and said, "It does make me feel like I won't fall." I said, "Great, I'll keep it handy for you then."

He continued to use the walker more and more, but it was a little big and heavy to get in the back of the SUV. I stopped at the medical supply store again and bought him a smaller one that was triangular shaped with a storage bag to carry things, like his books or newspaper. I added a cup holder so he could carry his water or milk and brought it home.

When I came in the house with it, his eyes lit up. "It's perfect with the bag attached in the middle, I can carry my books and stuff." He put it to use immediately, and the larger one went into a small storage area, just in case he wanted to use it again. Bill would sometimes use the larger walker if he thought he would need to sit down while he was walking to catch his breath or rest.

When Bill started using the walker more and more, his posture was getting so bad due to back pain that he leaned over and had the walker at arm's length. The correct walking position is head up, arms out, but with the walker held close. You are supposed to walk inside the walker. I would often tell him, "Your head is ahead of your feet." He would be leaning so far over that if he fell, he would fall headfirst, flat on his face. I could easily see this happening, so I generally stayed close so I could hang on to his belt at the back of his waist, just to keep him steady.

Another trick I learned, or I should say figured out, is that when it was impossible to use the walker due to space limitations, I would stand in front of him, and he would put his hands on my shoulders, and we would walk together with me in front. I was essentially the walker, but I had to warn him not to put all his weight on my shoulders, or I would fall with him if he went down.

The name of the smaller walker is a "Winnie." We named it Baby Winnie and the larger one Big Winnie. I would ask do you want "Baby Winnie or Big Winnie in the car?" He would choose which one he wanted depending on where we were going. I'd grab the one he asked for, fold it up and throw it into the back of the SUV.

Eventually, I would stop and buy Bill a wheelchair. He had several days of pain in his ankle and difficulty walking. I knew he would not want to use it much, but it was his birthday soon, and he wanted to go to a museum for the day. I knew he would never be able to walk the whole day.

The chair I bought was called a "transporter." It had smaller wheels than a wheelchair, which makes it a little lighter weight. Bill weighed over two-hundred pounds, so I was hoping it would make my job of pushing him easier. We would eventually buy another wheelchair, too, as it had bigger wheels which are supposed to make it easier to push, but it was heavier to get in the car.

We didn't use either wheelchair very often, but when we did, it made life a little better for Bill. Getting into the doctor's office or the hospital was quicker and easier with less pain when he used one of the wheelchairs. He never really liked sitting in them but would use one if I said he needed to because of the circumstances. He didn't like it when I had to push the wheelchair. He was very considerate of my back and didn't want me to get hurt.

The final and biggest investment we made was a three-wheeled scooter. We went to the medical supply store again, who, by now, loved us for all the items we had purchased there, and Bill gave one a try. It was my idea, of course, and he was hesitant but did think it was kind of fun to ride.

They are heavy but come apart, so you can get them in the back of the car if needed. I learned to take it apart and put it back together, but to this day, Bill has only used it to go around the corner of our neighborhood. On one of these trips, he crashed the scooter by hitting the curb at the wrong angle for the front wheel. If it had not been for several gardeners in the area that came running to help us, I don't think I would have gotten him off the pavement. This was scary for Bill, so he's never used it again, but it remains in the garage waiting patiently for the day he will use it more often, even if it's just in the house. I hoped it would be soon.

GI Bleed

Lesson: A Few Minutes of Deep Breathing Can Quell Anxiety

One quiet Saturday night at our house, we were watching a movie on TV and Bill seemed comfortable and looked well. He's not had any atrial fib for awhile, and he feels pretty good. He got up to go to the bathroom, and the cushion he had been sitting on was covered in blood. "Oh my God, this looks bad." I told him to go in the bathroom and wipe himself to check if he was still bleeding and to try and get an idea of how bad it was.

Gastrointestinal Bleeds, also known as a GI bleed, can be quite serious, or they can be as simple as a bleeding hemorrhoid. But when I looked at the cushion, I knew it was too much blood for a hemorrhoid. We had to get to the emergency room, even if Bill was saying, "I don't want to go!"

This happened about 7:00 p.m. I determined there was enough bleeding that it would require medical intervention. I decided to call the advice nurse to ask what to do first. The hold time time was over an hour, and I guessed the nurse would probably tell me to take him to the emergency room, so I hung up, and skipped this step. I gathered his belongings and equipment and ushered him out to the car, sat him in the passenger seat with a towel and a protective pad under his bottom and off we went.

By 8 p.m., we had arrived at the emergency room and have been checked in. It's the weekend when they are always very busy, and this night was no exception. For the first time in all our adventures to the emergency room, we have the same doctor we had on a previous visit. She had been pregnant the last time we saw her, and I asked her what she had. "You took care of Bill another time and you were pregnant, what did you have?"

She smiled and pulled out her phone and said, "Look at what I made!" A sweet-faced baby boy was in the picture. She then remembered us, and I knew that would help Bill get the best care. There is nothing better than having a previous encounter with a doctor, and they remember you to get the most attention.

She went over Bill's history and examined him. He was still actively bleeding, so an IV was started, and blood was drawn for lab work to see if his blood count was dropping. For the most part, it takes a while for a drop in hematocrit and hemoglobin after someone bleeds before it shows up in lab work, unless it is a significant bleed, most likely from trauma, then it shows up within thirty minutes or so.

Bill was not hemorrhaging, which was good, but a bleed like this is always concerning. He would be admitted, and his Pradaxa would be stopped. This was the most worrisome part of the night. He was not in atrial fib, but it is possible to form clots after stopping an anticoagulant like Pradaxa. It takes approximately one to two days for Pradaxa to be out of the system, but it is still risky as blood clots can form at any time after stopping the drug.

It took several hours to get Bill admitted. I had his CPAP machine in the car, so I brought it in, and since it was after midnight, he told me to go home. I was comfortable leaving him, so I drove home about 1:00 a.m. I woke up and called the hospital about 3:00 a.m. to find out what room they had put him in and to check on him. The nurse said, "He's fine, sleeping now." I knew from my nurse training that you never really report anything bad on the phone, so this answer, which was given often, I'm sure, still made me feel like I could go to sleep or try to sleep without worry.

I went back to the hospital about 8 a.m. the next day after I tried to get the stain out of the cushion. The furniture and cushions had been treated with an anti-stain spray to keep them clean when we purchased the chairs. I got the instructions out and washed the cushion with the soap they provided, and I was amazed that all the blood came out. Thankfully, there would be no memory of this hospital stay with a stained cushion I would have to throw away. I was hoping if this was so easy, the rest of the day with Bill would go well, too.

I was at the hospital by 9:00 a.m., and Bill was up and eating a little breakfast when I arrived. He was roaring that he had not slept all night. "It's too noisy and they keep waking me up to check my blood pressure." I said, "I'm sorry you haven't slept, why don't I turn the lights off now and you try to nap before the doctor comes in." I turned off the lights, and he closed his eyes.

I read while he napped, but it wouldn't last long because

a nurse came in or a lab technician came to draw blood, which got him all riled up again. When the doctor arrived later in the morning, Bill's first question was, "Why do they have to keep waking me up to take my blood pressure?" The doctor quietly said, "Well, you wouldn't want to take your car in to have it tuned up and not have them check the oil." I laughed out loud, I loved this answer, and it quieted Bill down right away.

Eventually, it was determined that Bill was no longer bleeding, and they would do a colonoscopy to check to see what had caused the bleeding. He was sent home, and the test would be done as an outpatient. I was relieved, and so was Bill, but the question uppermost in my mind was when to restart the Pradaxa they had stopped due to the bleeding.

Before we left the hospital, another doctor came in and told us to start the Pradaxa in four days if there was no more bleeding. I told him that I would take care of it. As this was a Sunday, I said, "I'll restart the medication on Wednesday." He said, "That's perfect."

I brought Bill home, and he slept for what seemed like days to catch up on the sleep he lost while in the hospital. On Monday, we got a call from the outpatient clinic to tell us the colonoscopy was scheduled for Thursday. I was told not to restart the Pradaxa until after the colonoscopy. I was getting worried this was too long to wait but didn't argue with the nurse. It wouldn't have done much good anyway.

Wednesday night, he began the prep for the test. When he began drinking the terrible tasting liquid required to clean out the bowel, he would look at me with very sad eyes and say, "Do I really have to do this?" I had to tell him, "Yes, you do, they have to find out what is making you bleed." He continued to drink the prep and finally stayed in the bathroom because he was getting so weak, walking back and forth from bedroom to bathroom was becoming too much for him.

That being done, Bill went to bed and was ready for the test the next day. I pushed him into the hospital in a wheelchair and got him to the outpatient surgery area for the test. I stayed in the waiting area in case of a problem, and they needed me. I read while the test was done.

The results were good. There was no more bleeding, just some polyps that needed to be taken care of. I took Bill home to sleep off the sedation they gave him for the test. Things were looking brighter, and I was breathing a little easier. When my anxiety ran rampant during these times, I could feel my neck and chest tighten like I couldn't get a full breath in my lungs. I was looking for more ways to relieve this feeling, and deep breaths became part of the answer.

There are many benefits to deep breathing, and I had to learn to take care of myself by practicing this technique more and more. I would sometimes forget, so I was once told by a therapist to put a rubber band around my wrist and snap it when I felt like I was being overwhelmed with anxiety. This also reminded me to take a deep breath.

The physical and emotional benefits of deep breaths are many. Here are just a few. The last one was very important as I was doing more and more caregiving, and I needed to stay well and curb my anxiety and hypervigilance.

Physical and Emotional Benefits from Deep Breathing:

- Reduces stress levels in your body
- Lowers your heart rate

- Lowers your blood pressure
- Reduces depression
- Better manages chronic pain
- Better regulates your body's reaction to stress and fatigue
- Reduces the possibility of burnout for caregivers

Once Bill returned home and began to feel better, after the sedation wore off, we settled into our routine again rather quickly. He was up on Friday, eating and reading the newspapers he normally would read every morning with no problems. I went about the day without further worry about this incident, catching up on chores I didn't get done while I had been busy at the hospital with Bill earlier in the week. Little did I know, or expect, that we would be back to the hospital the next day.

Stroke or TIA

Lesson: Don't Forget Communication Devices

I had signed up for a meditation class at the Lodge where we lived on the Saturday after Bill came home from the hospital after his colonoscopy. "I'm fine, go ahead to your class. Don't worry." He told me. It was just a two-hour class and ten minutes away. Bill felt he was well enough to run some errands and do some shopping. I did not want him to do too much without me in the car with him, but I felt I had to let him get back to his routine. I gave little thought to the idea that just because the sun was out, it didn't mean that rain could be on the horizon.

I had my iPhone with me, but I forgot to put my iWatch on that day. It didn't occur to me that we would turn off our phones in class, so I just left the house without thinking about it. If you aren't familiar with iPhones and iWatches, they are both Apple products. When your phone rings, you also get a signal on your watch. Even if your phone is off, the watch will respond to the call. You can see who is calling and decide if you are going to leave the room and take the call quietly or let it go to voicemail.

My class was quiet and peaceful and a great way to spend a Saturday morning after a stressful week. As I was walking to the car after class, I turned my phone on and saw there were two messages. One from Bill and one from a number I didn't recognize. Damn, why had I not worn my watch or left the phone on vibrate?

Message one from Bill: "I was at the library dumping the cardboard in the recycler and I think I'm having a stroke. My left hand and wrist aren't working. I'm home now and I'm going to call 9-1-1." My heart skipped a beat, and I took a huge deep breath.

Message two was from the fire department: "We have Bill in the ambulance, he's possibly had a stroke, he is doing fine. His left hand is affected for the most part, but he's fine, call me if you have questions." He left me a phone number.

I returned the call to the fire chief. "He's doing fine, I just heard over the radio calls that he's doing better. Don't rush to the hospital and get in an accident." I thanked him, and by then, I was home, had checked on the dog, and switched to Bill's car and headed for the hospital. I had to trade cars because if Bill was sent home he could not get in my small car.

I got to the hospital in about thirty minutes. I checked in at the front desk and was immediately sent to his room. When I walked in, he was talking to a nurse, and she was checking him for other signs of a stroke. They were discussing the fingers of his left hand that weren't working as they normally should, but he seemed to be in good spirits and was being well cared for. I took a deep breath and asked, "What happened?"

"Well, I decided to take the cardboard boxes to the library recycling bin and when I got there, my left hand just wasn't working. It felt kind of numb and my fingers weren't right, so I drove myself home and tried to call you, but you didn't have your phone, did you?" A little accusingly.

I answered "I did have it, but I had to shut it off for class. I'm sorry." He proceeded to tell me he called 9-1-1 for himself, got the dog in her crate, opened the front door, and sat in the living room and waited for the ambulance.

I felt so incredibly bad about this. I couldn't stop thinking of what a horrible person I was to leave him alone and have this happen to him. But my commonsense side told me, "I told him not to take the cardboard to the recycler, and he won't use a cell phone, and I just can't be there all of the time." I still felt bad about it, but we moved on with the day in the emergency room. My anxiety level was high, but as per my nature, the emergency room does not scare me. It's just a waiting game that one must play.

After several tests, blood work, a CT scan, and a few visits from the doctor, Bill would be admitted. It was determined this was not a full stroke, but what is called a "TIA," or Transient Ischemic Attack. My question to everyone was, "He was off his Pradaxa for almost a week, do you think that was the problem?" I wanted to curse at every doctor that walked in because this was so preventable if I had given him the Pradaxa sooner once they determined he was not hemorrhaging. It seemed this was my medical opinion, but no one elses.

A TIA is a "warning stroke" that occurs when a blood clot blocks an artery for a short time. The only difference between a stroke and TIA is that with a TIA, the blockage is usually temporary. The symptoms occur rapidly and last a relatively short time. Unlike a stroke, when a TIA is over, there's no permanent injury to the brain. There's no way to tell if symptoms of a stroke will lead to a TIA or a major stroke.

The American Heart Association uses the word "FAST" to remember the signs of a stroke.

> **F-ace Drooping:** Does one side of the face droop, or is it numb? Ask the person to smile.
>
> **A-rm Weakness:** Is one arm weak or numb? Ask the person to raise both arms.
>
> **S-peech Difficulty:** Is speech slurred? Is the person unable to speak or hard to understand?
>
> **T-ime to call 9-1-1:** If someone shows any of these symptoms, even if the symptoms go away, call 9-1-1 and get the person to the hospital immediately.

Be sure to check the time, so you know when the first symptoms appeared to report to the doctor.

Other symptoms to watch for include:

- Blindness in one or both eyes or double vision
- Vertigo or loss of balance or coordination

Bill's hand and arm numbness or slight paralysis was already resolving, but he would need to have some more testing done to make sure another TIA or stroke was not on the horizon. Also, to see if there was any permanent damage to his brain. Eventually, the doctor would order some physical therapy for him when he was sent home to make sure he had full use of his hand again.

At about 5:00 p.m., I decided I had to go home and get the CPAP machine. I did not learn my lesson on this ER visit, as I was in such a hurry. I grabbed something to eat, fed the dog, who was very upset herself because she had not been out for a while, and was waiting for someone, anyone, to come home and feed her. I was back at the hospital by 7:00 p.m.

Bill was now comfortably situated in a private room that was quiet and seemed relaxing for him. The nurses were pleasant and following the doctor's orders for Bill's medications, lab work, and tests. I was feeling secure with just staying for a while, going home, and leaving him alone for the night.

The next day, I arrived early, and we were waiting patiently, well sort of, for the neurologist to arrive. Why do doctor's visits always seem to happen later in the day? Of course, this was Sunday, and it was understandable that the doctors would operate on a slightly different schedule.

I had notified Bill's daughters that he was in the hospital, and they both stopped by for a short visit. A close friend came by to bring him a book and check on him, as well. He was in good spirits and looked "healthy" while resting in his hospital bed. Everyone expressed the thought that he would be fine because he looked so good. The doctor finally arrived.

He told Bill that it looked like the TIA was more from high cholesterol than a blood clot. Stopping the Pradaxa had not been the issue. There was a new medication to be started to lower his cholesterol, and that would be done immediately. He also wanted to order a scan of Bill's heart to make sure there were no blood clots lurking in any of the chambers because he had been off the Pradaxa for almost a week since the GI bleed. The doctor ordered the Pradaxa to be restarted, and Bill would be able to go home the next day.

Bill told the doctor, "I want to go home today!" I suggested he stay so I could go home and get some rest before he came home, and he tells the doctor, "She just wants to have her boyfriend over, that's why she doesn't want me home." I was devastated and could not believe he could say such a cruel thing. I left the room in tears.

The doctor came out of the room and told me, "I'll order the scan of his heart, but I'm not sure it can be done on a Sunday." I said, "That's fine, whenever it can be done will work." I went back into Bill's room. My feelings were very hurt, but I didn't say a word. The nurse came into the room and said, "The scan looks like it will be tomorrow." It was about 3:00 p.m., and I was so tired I could barely keep my eyes open. "I'm going home for a while, to feed the dog, and get something to eat, I'll come back later." Bill said, a little unhappy at my leaving, "Okay, see you later."

When I walked into the house, the phone was ringing, and I ran to answer it. Without even saying "Hello," Bill says, "Come and get me, they are going to do the scan this afternoon." I asked when, he said, "I don't know."

I fed the dog, picked up my purse, got back in the car, and drove the thirty minutes back to the hospital. When I arrived, they had not even started the scan yet. I waited over two hours for them to finish and get Bill ready for discharge. Then, I was sent to the pharmacy to pick up his new prescription. I was exhausted but tried to remain calm when I so badly wanted to say, "I could have stayed home a while and then come back." Bill wanted to go home, and that was the end of the discussion.

We got home, and I fixed some dinner, and we went to bed early. I was still stinging from what Bill said to the doctor about my not wanting to take him home, but I stayed quiet about it until Bill was rested and felt a bit better. A few days later, I asked him, "Why would you say something so cruel about my not wanting to bring you home?" He said he didn't remember saying it. Well, now I was in fear that the TIA had affected his brain, although they are not supposed to. Memory loss was becoming an issue with him. A new battle had begun!

Cognitive Decline

Lesson: "Honey" Makes Life Sweeter

Bill began to forget a lot of things, I wanted to say everything, but some days his memory was better than other days. He would ask the same questions over and over. "What are we doing today?" "Who is coming today?" "Where are you going?" The last question asked the most frequently. I would tell him what was happening every day in the morning, but partway through the day, he would often ask, "What is happening, is anybody coming today?"

This began to worry me, so I made a doctor's appointment for him. He generally wasn't feeling well anyway, so I thought it was a good time to have him see his primary care physician (PCP). When I called the nurse, I told her what was going on, so she made the appointment for a longer span of time, knowing that the doctor may need longer to see him. She also said, "We'll do a cognitive test, and that takes a while too."

I was curious what a cognitive test was, so again, I referred to our health plan's website and the internet. I found the following information on the Center for Disease Control and Prevention website. The reason the CDC is looking into cognitive decline is that with our aging population, it is becoming a public health crisis. And here, I just thought it was a problem at my house or in my retirement community. I was wrong, of course, and should have known better.

Subjective cognitive decline (SCD) is the self-reported experience of more frequent confusion and memory loss by a patient. It is one of the earliest symptoms of Alzheimer's disease and related dementia. It is a health crisis because it has implications for living with and managing chronic disease and performing activities like cooking, cleaning, and self-care.

Cognition is a process in the brain that is a combination of the ability to learn, remember and make judgments. This causes a profound impact on individuals and their overall health and well-being. Cognitive decline can range from mild cognitive impairment to dementia. Dementia, on the other hand, is a decline so severe it interferes with daily life. Alzheimer's is the more common form of dementia.

Some cognitive decline happens as a person ages, but frequently forgetting routine tasks is not a normal part of aging and can cause problems with an individual's activities of daily living (ADL). These are cooking, finances, self-care, medical appointment management, and medications. It is thought that with some education and modifications, some of these issues can be managed for the health and well-being of the patient.

When we visited the doctor, she did a full exam of Bill, including reflexes, eye movements, walking, and balance. Bill could not do the walking and balance test because of his bad ankle and weakness. She then told us, "Someone will be in to do a mental status test in a few minutes." We said, "OK," and waited. We had no idea what to expect. Bill asked me, "What does that mean?" I had to say, "I don't know, let's wait and see."

A nurse came in with a paper that she read questions from to test Bill's memory. One of the tests was, "Name as many animals as you can in thirty seconds." He hesitated and could name a few and then lost his concentration. There were more basic questions like, "Who is the president?" He named the last president, not the current one. "What is the day of the week?" He looked at me, and I said, "I can't help you, I'm sorry." There were some other basic questions that he did well with. The real problem came when the nurse handed him the paper and asked him to draw a clock with the time 10:50 on it.

Bill drew the circle and put the numbers in from nine to twelve, but did not get the hands of the clock in the correct position. I honestly had to think about how to do this, as well. He knew it was wrong but didn't know how to fix it, so he handed the paper to the nurse. "How did I do?" he asked.

"You did fine." She said, "I'll have the doctor look at it and she will come back and give you the score." She left the room, and Bill asked again, "How did I do?" I told him, "I think you did fine, you missed a question or two, but don't worry about it."

The doctor came in and told Bill he had a score of 21. "What does that mean?" Bill asked. She said the test is scored based on the highest being 30 points. This means you have some mild dementia." His eyes got big, he looked at me, and she continued to explain. 'We'll continue to watch this and see you in six months for another test." I asked, "Is there any medication he can start for this?" She answered, "Not yet. We'll see how he does in six months.

I asked to see the scoring criteria on the paper while she continued to talk to Bill. Here is what the scores mean on the test.

The test has a maximum score of 30 points. The scores are generally grouped as follows:

25-30 points: Normal Cognition

21-24 points: Mild Dementia

10 to 20 points: Moderate Dementia

9 points or less: Severe Dementia

I could see that Bill's score was getting close to moderate dementia, and we would really need to watch this and report to the doctor any further worsening of symptoms. Bill had also lost about six pounds, and his blood pressure was low. The doctor told me, "Take his blood pressure everyday and let me know if it stays low and if he loses more weight."

We now had evidence that Bill was beginning to suffer some memory impairment. Bill could remember who he sat next to in first grade, but current memories failed him. It seemed the old memories have remained in his head better than the new ones. He frequently asked where I was going several times before I went anywhere, even though I had already told him several times that day and probably the day before. This is common with patients who have dementia.

Bill reads all the time, it's his only entertainment except for the news on the television. Two newspapers a day and many books always sit by his chair. The doctor told him to do games like sudoku or crossword puzzles to keep his dementia from getting worse. Keeping the brain active can decrease the decline or slow it down. Bill told her, "I read all of the time, I should be okay." The doctor said, "No, reading is an old skill you learned so it's part of the old memory bank. Reading won't really help." Bill has never picked up a puzzle, and I doubt he will.

Bill was never mean or hard to live with when his memory began to fail him. He remained the sweet, gentle guy I married. But my attitude had to change. I was answering the same questions over and over, and sometimes, this caused impatience on my side of the conversation. The most obvious impairment for Bill, besides his memory, was using the three remote controls it took to run the television. He just couldn't hit the right button no matter how hard he tried.

I found that if I only covered one thing at a time in a question or statement, I was much better off in communicating with Bill. Too many things going on at one time were distracting to him. He loved to talk about the old days, and it was hard to keep him focused on current questions and issues. I would sometimes have to bring him back to the present time by joking with him and saying, "Could we stick to the twenty-first century please?" This would make him think a bit, but it didn't always bring him back to the present day if he was stuck on an old story.

Since he had been an attorney, I would also say, "Your honor, would you please instruct the witness to answer the question?" This made him smile and would bring him back to the question I had asked. But only sometimes. The sad thing is all the old memories were at the top of his brain or at the forefront, so they always came first, it seemed, when he was talking. And of course, they got repeated frequently, especially the happiest ones.

Sometimes when I would talk to him, I would preface the sentence with the word, "Honey." I never used this kind of endearment, so it felt extra special when I did. It seemed to soften the "blow" of what I was about to say or get his attention. When I was having a hard time communicating with Bill, I would sit in front of him and say, "Honey," and continue the sentence or question, or ask my question and end with "Honey." It seemed to work well and get the desired attention.

Here are ten tips for communicating with the cognitively declined individual from the Caregiver.org website that I found very helpful:

• Set a positive mood for the interaction.
    Speak in a positive, pleasant, and respectful manner. Use facial expressions, tone of voice, and physical touch to help convey your message and show affection.

• Get the person's attention.
    Limit distractions and noise. Turn off the TV and move to quiet surroundings, if necessary. Sit next to the person, make eye contact, and use non-verbal cues like touch to help keep the person focused.

• State your message clearly.
    Use simple words and sentences. Speak slowly and in a reassuring tone. Don't raise your voice. Lower it instead. If the person doesn't understand, repeat the message in the exact words, and speak distinctly.

If there is still no understanding, rephrase the question.

- Ask simple questions.

  Ask one question at a time, those with a yes or no answer work best. Refrain from asking questions that give too many choices. Use visual prompts and cues to help clarify the question and guide the response.

- Listen with your eyes, ears, and heart.

  Be patient while waiting for a reply. Give the person time to think of the answer, and then suggest words if you think you can help them find the word they are looking for. Always listen for meaning and feelings that might underlie the words.

- Break down activities into a series of steps.

  Encourage your loved ones to do what they can. Gently remind them of steps they might have forgotten and assist with the steps they can no longer accomplish. Use visual clues to help the person remember.

- Use distraction or redirect the person if they get upset.

  Change the subject or the environment if the person is distracted or upset. Let them know you are aware of their feelings. "I see you are a little distracted, I'm sorry, let's go do something else." Make it something they enjoy, like TV, music or reading.

- Always respond with affection and reassurance.

  A person with dementia may feel confused, anxious, and unsure of themselves, getting reality confused with the past. They may recall things that never occurred. Don't correct them. Stay focused on the feelings they are expressing. Sometimes touching, hugging, and praise can reassure the person and help them respond appropriately.

- Remembering the good old days.

  Remembering the past is often soothing to the patient, the times when they were the happiest. Remembering what happened forty-five minutes ago will be hard, but remembering what happened forty-five years ago is much easier for them. Try and avoid questions that rely on short-term memory.

- Maintain a sense of humor.

  Use humor when you can, but don't make fun of the person or use humor at their expense. People with dementia often are delighted to laugh along with you.

I'd like to add one more personal item to this list. Don't take offense at some of the things that are said by someone suffering from cognitive decline. Sometimes things come out of their mouth without any thought. These can be rude, thoughtless things they would never have said in the past, like Bill's comment to the doctor that I didn't want to take him home because I wanted to have my boyfriend over.

Bill constantly lives in the past. He had a great career and a great time growing up, and much of what he remembers is of his childhood, life with his mother, law school, and his work. Very few memories are of our life together, and I don't seem to be a part of any his memories. I mentioned this to him one day, "Your memories don't seem to include any of the wonderful things we have done in our life together." He looked at me in total shock, "What, I don't? Maybe it's because you are still here and take care of me." I had no response, but it did make him think. It didn't change anything. He still only talks about the old memories before I knew him, unless it's our anniversary and we talk about the arch in the backyard swaying in the wind. At least he still has good memories of that special day.

Another odd thing that has happened with Bill's memory failing is he doesn't turn out any lights anymore. If I left my office to check on him while he was resting, I have found the kitchen, dining room, and living room lights were left on after he was in those rooms. This happens a lot during the day, the lights don't even need to be on, but he seems to turn them on every time he walks into a room. When I discovered all the lights are on, I walked through the house and turned them off and went back to what I was doing. If I mentioned this to him, he wouldn't remember he had turned them on, and it just wasn't necessary to bother him with the issue.

Calling an Ambulance

Lesson: If You Think It's Necessary - Call

I was beginning to feel like I was constantly making the decision to call an ambulance. When Bill called one for himself when he had his TIA, it was very unusual, but I wasn't home, so he had taken charge.

When to call an ambulance is always a difficult decision. Waiting too long can make the emergency worse, so don't second guess yourself for too long. You'll ask yourself, "Should I drive my loved one to the hospital?" "What if something happens halfway to the hospital, and I can't get them there fast enough?" "Is it expensive to call an ambulance?" "Will the ambulance drivers think I'm stupid?" If you feel your loved one is in trouble and you can't handle it, "CALL!"

Here are some of the instances when calling an ambulance is appropriate, and it might help guide you in your decision. These are just some of the reasons. There are many other times when you will feel it is safer for an ambulance to come, rather than to drive the person yourself.

- The person's condition is life-threatening. This could include chest pain, difficulty breathing, sudden confusion, or altered mental status. These conditions could be signs of stroke, heart attack, or a related condition and require immediate attention.

- Someone is choking and needs the abdominal thrusts known as the Heimlich maneuver or black blows to dislodge something in the wind-pipe, such as food or a pill.

- Massive bleeding from a wound.

- Moving the patient may further the individual's condition, such as in a fall or a car accident.

- If you are alone, and you become too weak and unable to get yourself to the emergency room or have no one to call to help you.

Ambulance drivers are some of the nicest people you will ever meet. They will never criticize your reason's for calling. The ambulance personnel can help you make the decision as to whether your loved one's illness or symptoms require a trip to the ER by ambulance or private car.

They will also help with falls, getting the person off the floor, check their blood pressure, and put them on a heart monitor to possibly determine the cause of the fall. If it's decided the patient is not in serious condition, they can recommend that you take them to the hospital or urgent care. If there is doubt as to the cause of the fall they will take the patient to the hospital.

Don't ever worry that you are taking the ambulance and personnel from other people who might need them more.

There are always several companies within an area, even if from another county. During the Covid pandemic, we were asked not to call an ambulance unless it was for one of the above reasons as they were in short supply to get Covid patients to the hospital.

In my county, if you dial 9-1-1, the fire department will arrive first and then the ambulance. If the fire department determines they can handle the problem, they can cancel the ambulance. All personnel have some medical training so the fire department can read the heart monitor and take blood pressure as well as the ambulance personnel. This could be different where you live, so you might want to investigate.

If you live in a rural area, the response time for a 9-1-1 call can vary considerably. If your fire department is a volunteer department, that may also change the response time. You should still call for help but be prepared to wait and possibly offer some emergency first aid to the victim as well.

This is a good case where you might find it beneficial to learn CPR. It's a good skill to learn no matter where you live, and if you took the course several years ago, things remain pretty much the same in that rescue breathing is given along with chest compressions.

If you feel you are qualified to start CPR on a person without a heartbeat and/or who is no longer breathing, call 9-1-1 first and then start CPR, the operator can assist you with directions for checking the patient and beginning CPR if you are unsure.

To learn CPR, go to www.redcross.org for more information. You can also learn to do the Heimlich maneuver to aid someone who is choking.

In the case of someone who has fallen and needs help to get up, here in my city, there is a special number to call, so you don't activate the EMS (Emergency Medical System) or the 9-1-1 system. You call this number if you just need help getting someone off the floor, and they don't need medical attention. If help arrives and determines the fall is more serious, they can activate the Emergency Medical System and get the rest of the medical personnel needed to take care of the patient.

If the patient has the "I've fallen and I can't get up button" around their neck or on their wrist, or the module by the bed, you can decide with the provider as to who they call if the patient activates the EMS system by using the button.

I have arranged with the people who answer the phone for our system that if I am not at home, they are to call me and tell me what the situation is before an ambulance is called. This is the reason I never left the house without my phone, even to walk the dog. If Bill were to press the button for help, I would get a call and then have to decide who should be called for emergency help or if no call should be made, depending on his condition.

If you make the decision to drive your loved one to the hospital yourself and something happens on the way there, like they fall unconscious, have vomiting that won't stop, chest pain, shortness of breath, a headache that is suddenly much worse, excessive bleeding or excruciating abdominal pain. (These are just a few examples.) Pull over to a well-lit area if it's dark, a shopping center, or an easily accessed area if you can get there quickly and dial 9-1-1 from there.

You can tell the 9-1-1 dispatcher where you are so the

ambulance can find you. Turn on the emergency flashers of your car, and if a police officer sees you, he would likely stop. Do not leave the patient in the car and go looking for help! You need to be there when help arrives so you can tell the emergency personnel what is happening and the medical history of the patient.

If your loved one goes to the hospital in an ambulance, the ambulance personnel will generally recommend that you give the hospital staff some time to settle the patient and assess the situation before you rush to the emergency room. You cannot ride along with the patient, so you will need to take some deep breaths, gather your belongings and items from the list below, and get there slowly. In most cases, you won't be able to see the patient until the emergency personnel has settled them in, taken vital signs, and perhaps a doctor has been in for a visit.

I have found that by the time I have the dog settled, maybe I had to get dressed, called friends or family, and calmed down, by the time I got to the ER, they were just about ready for me to go in and stay with Bill. Of course, during the pandemic, you weren't allowed in to see your loved one at all. Thankfully, that was over for a short time, but now the Covid rules apply again, and you can't go into the emergency room with your loved one. I hope this is over soon. It's agonizing to sit outside and wonder what is happening.

Here are some recommendations for making a trip to the emergency room as comfortable as possible for both you and the patient. I've learned many a lesson about leaving the house in a hurry and forgetting some of the most important items, like the CPAP machine or shoes for Bill. It always seemed that it was about 2:00 a.m. when I needed to make the drive home to get the items, which I shouldn't have forgotten in the first place.

What to Take to the Emergency Room:

- Medical cards and ID
- List of medications for patient
- CPAP or any other equipment the patient might need
- Medication for yourself if there might be a long wait
- Your phone with a contact list, if none, your address book
- Phone charger
- Tablet with charger
- Money or ATM card for food or coffee
- Clothes for the patient, especially shoes, for when they are discharged
- Puzzles or word games to do while waiting
- Something to read: A book or an e-reader with a book on it and a charging cord, magazine, or newspaper.
- If you have a pet, get them situated, and be sure you have someone to feed them and let them out if you are delayed
- Sweater or jacket. Emergency rooms are traditionally cold, and you may be out in the middle of the night and need something warm to wear.

Calling an ambulance will always be a difficult decision with an uncertain ending. Staying calm and giving the ambulance and hospital personnel as much information as you can will make the visit go as smoothly as possible. Remember, all medical staff are well trained and need you to be there for support and love. Let them do their jobs and try and stay as positive and calm as possible.

Taking Charge

Lesson: Power of Attorney and Advanced Health Care Directives

As Bill became weaker and weaker, I was left with more to do. It all came about slowly, as I began doing more errands, banking, shopping, and household chores, and before I knew it, I was doing them all. It was a slow progression into the many things I had helped with before and now what I was totally responsible for. When two people are working together to do the household chores, planning, and shopping, it is work, but it can be fun. When one person takes over everything, it can become overwhelming.

Bill loved to grocery shop, and I would go with him when he did the shopping just to "go along for the ride." I would help find the items on the list and put them in the cart, but he picked out the meats and vegetables. No more! I was in charge and would have to learn to do it all.

I learned to fulfill every request for food or treats, especially when Bill began to lose weight and did not eat as well as he used to. I became quite familiar with the three local grocery stores and learned that shopping isn't too bad, especially when I learned to shop online and then picked up the groceries.

Eventually, Bill quit carrying his wallet as well, so if he went to the store with me, I always took care of checking out and paying. I also did this at restaurants, until one day I realized that he might want to take care of the bill because it was "his job," more or less. I didn't want to take everything away from him until he told me he was ready.

We didn't go out often, mostly for special occasions. On our anniversary, we went to a lovely restaurant for lunch, and Bill didn't leave a tip for the waitress. He thought they had added the tip on automatically. She was so kind to us that I wanted to go back to the restaurant and apologize. This error meant the decision was made; I would pay the checks from now on.

Once Bill was forced to give up driving, I took over that job as well. The thing is, I had a small sports car, and he had an SUV. He could not get in my car, so when we needed to go somewhere, it had to be in the SUV. It had a large trunk area to hold his walker or wheelchair as well. It was the reason we bought the car.

If I got rid of my car, we would have had more room in the garage, and it might then be easier for Bill to get into the SUV, but I still wasn't interested in selling it. We could have managed just fine with one car, but I didn't want to get rid of mine. Eventually, it would happen, but I loved that little car, and I was just not ready to give it up.

At some point, I would probably turn both cars in for something I could drive comfortably when I was alone, maybe a hybrid or electric car since I didn't go very far anymore. This, of course, would all depend on whether I moved from our large home to something smaller or assisted living when I was once alone. I wasn't ready to think about all of this yet, but it seemed I thought or worried about it all the time. At this point, I was only removing Bill's name from the title of the SUV, which would make it easier to sell later when he might not be available to sign.

I would switch between the two cars depending on my errands. If it was for a large grocery order I took the SUV, and for my fun little errands where I didn't need a lot of cargo space because my trunk was small, I took my car. Each car got a turn at some point during the week, yet neither car had very much mileage. I was responsible for taking both cars in for maintenance as well. This wasn't really a horrible job, just time-consuming. Both cars came from great dealerships where they served coffee and had nice places to sit and wait.

Eventually, I would take care of everything in the house as well. I hired many people to do maintenance around the house and a new gardener. I would always have them meet Bill and let him be part of the decisions I was making, but he, most of the time, really didn't care. He was writing the checks for their services, so I thought he should be involved in the decision as well as have some say in what was going on in the house. He was tired and really didn't feel well, so just let me go ahead with whatever I thought was right. I was grateful for this as it made it easier to do these jobs when there was no discussion.

I also had to take over the pill distribution because after we moved back to California, Bill was sleeping even more than usual. We went to see his doctor, who ordered some blood tests to check his thyroid. It revealed that Bill had a very low thyroid. "Bill, you have the lowest thyroid I have ever seen, no wonder you are so tired, are you taking your pills?"

No response from Bill. The doctor checked his pharmacy page, and it showed Bill had not refilled the thyroid medication for over a year. When I found out that he only took this pill occasionally, I guessed he was doing the same with all his other medications. Low thyroid makes one very tired and sleepy, and this was part of the answer to his long naps.

Every Saturday, I refilled the daily pill reminders with the day and time on the small lid of each square section. I would fill his pill reminder for two weeks. I didn't let him put the pills in the container anymore as he would often not fill the container for the right day and time or leave out pills. He didn't do this on purpose but would get tired and forget what pills he had already put in the container. I put his pill container in the kitchen, so I wouldn't forget to remind him, or he would see them and hopefully remember to take them himself.

Every morning I would bring in Bill's newspapers, set his pills in a little glass container next to them, and that would be his subtle reminder to take them. At 4 p.m., I would say, "Take your pills." I would get them out of the pill reminder container, get a fresh glass of water, and he would take his afternoon pills. This way, I was sure he was getting all his medication, and I wouldn't have to be counting his pills every day. Every now and then, he would miss a pill, but I usually kept a close eye on them, so this didn't happen often. "Take your pills" became a mantra at our house.

Bill continued to write the checks for the bills. I told him

I would take over, but he managed the checkbook just fine, so I didn't feel I needed to take the job away from him yet. The time was coming, as he had made a couple of mistakes in the checkbook, and I would have to quietly remind him to pay the taxes, etc. When he got too tired, it was not a good time to write checks.

Again, my taking over everything all at once was not only a lot of work for me but very difficult for Bill. He had lost so much already; it just didn't seem fair to snatch everything out of his hands at one time. Eventually, he would no longer carry his wallet, his ID was in my purse, and his credit and debit card would be canceled. This made fewer cards to worry about, and I only had to carry mine because I did all the banking and making purchases at stores and restaurants.

It was clear Bill was losing his independence. I was getting more and more responsibility, which I didn't mind, but the best way we could handle it was to just let it happen. There was no way to stop it, so we just had to live with it. The changes were slow in coming, and eventually, my being responsible for everything just fell into place. There was no choice, it just had to be that way. We then made the decision that I would have Bill's Power of Attorney, we would be sure his Advance Care Directive was up to date, and we would add a new form called POLST.

- Power of attorney, or POA, gives permission to another person, known as your agent, to act on your behalf in legal matters.
- It can be a general power of attorney, General POA, granting broad power over your affairs.

- It can be a special power of attorney, Special POA, allowing your agent power only over specific situations.
  - It includes writing checks, signing official documents, or handling other legal dealings.
  - Your agent does not need to be a lawyer. It can be your spouse or any person over age 18 you choose.
- You can also choose to make a durable power of attorney, meaning your agent's powers remain in effect if you become incompetent or incapable of handling your affairs.

Getting a power of attorney is a big decision. We chose to get one as I was taking over more and more of the duties and felt it was important if Bill were to become incapacitated that I could continue taking care of our finances and make all decisions needed without any fuss or legal issue. If you choose to initiate a power of attorney, you can prepare the document yourself; you can even find the forms online. You do not have to use a lawyer.

We also had in Bill's medical record an advanced health care directive. It is the best way to make sure your wishes are followed regarding your health, if you are unable to speak for yourself, by appointing another person to be your health care "agent." This person will have the legal authority to make decisions about your medical care if you become unable to make decisions for yourself. Your doctor must abide by your wishes when this form is signed by you and filed in your medical record.

The final form we had at home was called a POLST form. It is bright pink, and we were told to place it on the refrigerator, where an ambulance driver would look for it. POLST means Physician Orders for Life-Sustaining Treatment.

Your physician must sign this form after you have checked the type of treatment you would want if you became ill and an ambulance needs to take you to the hospital. It is in lieu of your medical record because they don't have it available. This directive must be followed and is in complement to your advance directive but does not replace it.

The ambulance driver would take it with them when they transported the patient. It is their "orders" as to how to treat or not treat the patient in the ambulance.

There are three areas that are addressed on the form:

A: Two choices:
    1. Attempt resuscitation-CPR.
    2. Do not attempt resuscitation-CPR.
B: There are three choices for treatment:
    1. Full Treatment: the primary goal is to prolong life by all medically effective means.
    2. Selective Treatment: the goal is to treat medical conditions while avoiding burdensome measures.
    3. Comfort-Focused Treatment: the goal is to maximize comfort only.
C: Three choices for Artificially Administered Nutrition:
    1. Long-term artificial nutrition, including a feeding tube.
    2. Trial period of artificial nutrition, including a feeding tube.

3. No artificial means of nutrition, including a feeding tube.

D: Information and signatures:

The doctor and the patient sign the form. A copy of it is then placed in the patient's medical record.

If a section is left blank, it is implied that the patient wants the full listed treatment.

I sent Bill to the hospital in an ambulance one night when he had chest pain, and the EMTs took the form with them, as they are supposed to, yet it was not given back to Bill when it was time for discharge. That meant that we had to go to the doctor to have a new form filled out. At first, I thought it was just a lot of trouble, but it turned out to be a good idea. The patient's condition may have changed while they were in the hospital, and new decisions might need to be made.

All these forms will give you peace of mind while dealing with a long-term illness. They allow the patient to help make the decisions while they are feeling well enough to take all ramifications into consideration. For the caregiver, it helps them know they are following the patient's desires when it comes to health care, finances, as well as death and dying.

The Nasal Surgery Crash

Lesson: You Never Know How Strong You Are Until It's Your Only Choice

Bill had suffered from miserable sinus infections and the pain they caused for several months. I finally got him to go to see his primary care doctor, who sent him to an ear, nose, and throat specialist, now known as a head and neck surgeon. We waited a month for the appointment while Bill continued to suffer.

The doctor put a little scope into Bill's nose called a nasal endoscope so she could look up into the sinus cavity. What she saw showed up on a small screen while she was moving the probe around inside the nose and sinus area. I had no experience with this, but even I could tell there was something wrong inside his nose because it looked swollen, red, and had what looked like "yuk" inside the sinus cavity.

The doctor finished her exam and told him his sinuses were very badly infected, and he needed surgery to clean them out. Bill refused the surgery. "I don't want another surgery, I'll be fine." That's what he said to any type of treatment offered to him at the time, I'm afraid. We went home with orders for him to do sinus washes twice a day with salt water.

Sinus washes are miserable, I knew this would be hard for him, but he said he would try. If you've never done one, here is a brief description: Use sterile water mixed with a packet of pure salt that comes with a device called a "Neti" pot. The pot looks like a small teapot, or there are other devices that you squeeze to get the water into the nose that look like a syringe or a soft-sided bottle.

The first step is to create a saline solution. Typically, this is done by mixing warm, sterile water with pure salt, known as sodium chloride, to create an isotonic solution. You would then stand with your head over a sink or in the shower and tilt your head to one side. Pour or squeeze the salt solution slowly into one nostril and allow the fluid to run out the other nostril.

Repeat for the other side of the nose, tilting your head in the opposite direction. It all sounds simple enough, but you cough, sputter and spit while you have saltwater pouring out your nose and hopefully not down your throat. It's messy, and you blow your nose quite a bit when finished to get all the mucous out. I knew Bill would not like this. But then again, I wouldn't like it either.

As I predicted, he did the rinses for about two weeks and then quit. The doctor saw him again, two weeks after he quit the rinses, and told him he would still have to have surgery to clean out his sinus cavity. She told him, "The chronic infection could lead to serious problems like a brain abscess, meningitis, or infection in the bones."

Bill finally agreed to the surgery, but he was not happy

about it. It's a hard surgery to recover from, and the sinus rinses would need to be done twice daily again. His oldest daughter had the surgery done and told him it was a miserable experience. That was not at all helpful in getting him to do the surgery. Bill continued to feel awful. The infection, I believe, was taking a toll on him.

Our health insurance required a medical doctor to examine a patient before any surgery was done. I was afraid that Bill was in such poor shape that a doctor would not approve the surgery. I was almost hoping this, as I thought the recovery would be harder since he was already not feeling well and getting weaker.

I took Bill to the appointment, and he had a physical and an EKG; the doctor asked him a few questions and then approved the surgery. I wanted to go in and ask, "What are you thinking, the man can barely walk and his oxygen level is only in the low 90s?" But then again, I couldn't really do that. Or could I? I second-guessed myself on this for a long time, what if I had spoken up? Would it have changed anything? It would not have changed his final diagnosis, but maybe it wouldn't have been so traumatic getting it.

We were given the paperwork with the requirements for getting him ready for surgery, and they would call with the day and time later. We went home, and Bill went to bed. He stayed there almost continuously until his surgery date, about ten days later.

The day of the surgery arrived, and I was to get Bill to the hospital and admitted at 10:00 a.m. He was so weak that I had to push him in a wheelchair from the parking lot to the hospital and up to surgery admitting. He got checked in, and all was well until they had to weigh him. He could not stand on the scale. It was obvious to me that he was not in very good shape to go to surgery, but the nurses carried on with the orders, and he was made ready to go into surgery. I said a huge prayer that he would survive and gave him a hug, and sent him on his way.

About an hour after he went into surgery, I got a phone call from the doctor. I began to shake; I knew this wasn't good news. I was in the cafeteria and found the closest chair to sit down. "We had to stop the surgery, after Bill was intubated, he desaturated to forty so anesthesia called the surgery." She knew I knew this meant his oxygen level dropped to forty, while they were giving him 100 percent oxygen down the tube in his throat, and the surgery had not even gotten started.

She continued, "They are moving him to the recovery room, take your time and they will let you come in and see him and talk to the anesthesiologist." I said, "I'm just downstairs, I'll be right there."

When I arrived at the surgery waiting room, the coordinator that lets people in and out of the recovery room to see their loved ones would not let me in. Without getting too crazy with him, I said, "The doctor just called, his surgery was canceled, and I need to talk to the anesthesiologist." He finally let me in. When I got back to Bill's cubicle, it was a whirlwind. Several doctors and nurses were taking care of him. The anesthesiologist came to talk to me and told me. "He "coded" in surgery, and we had to start CPR." This was very serious.

The anesthesiologist told me he thought Bill had a pulmonary embolus, so he called off the surgery. A pulmonary embolus is a blood clot in the lung. It's very dangerous and can be quite deadly. The doctor had this happen to another patient in a similar situation, and he didn't want to risk continuing surgery because the other patient had died.

Bill had a CT scan to see if there were blood clots, thankfully there were none, and several other tests to determine why he quit breathing. Nothing was definite, and no one knew for sure what had happened. After several hours in the recovery room, he was admitted for more tests to determine the cause of his low oxygen level.

After Bill was settled in a room, I was heading home to feed the dog, so I could return for the evening. My cell phone rang as I was just stepping out the door of the hospital. It was Bill's oldest daughter. "You always let me know what happens with Dad right away, why haven't I heard from you?" She sounded a little angry with me.

I took a deep breath and told her what had happened. It sounded like she was having a panic attack with rapid breathing and gasping for air. I tried to calm her down as best I could over the phone. She wasn't at home, but on a camping trip with her husband, so she had to accept what I told her. I couldn't help her understand over the phone that he was all right for now. She would not be able to get to the hospital to see Bill even if she wanted to, so she had to accept what I told her. I tried to reassure her he would be fine, yet I wasn't sure of this myself.

When I returned to the hospital that evening, Bill was sitting up in bed and looked pretty good. He had oxygen running through a nasal cannula, and his PO2 levels were monitored constantly with the little device that looked like an old-fashioned clothespin on his finger. (PO2 means partial pressure of oxygen in the blood, pronounced pee-oh-too.) I spoke with his nurse, who thought he was doing well enough to go home the next day, but we would have to wait to see how he did during the night. I left the hospital feeling confident all was going to be okay.

I went back to the hospital the next day and waited to talk to the doctor to find out if Bill was going to be discharged home or if they would do more tests while he was there. The doctor came to visit about 11:00 a.m., and we talked about his drop in oxygen that so far, no one could explain the cause.

I told the doctor that his oxygen level was low even before the attempted surgery, and I was concerned that they should never have even tried to take him to the operating room. She told the nurses, "Walk him around with the PO2 monitor on his finger and see what his oxygen drops to when he walks."

Within just a few steps, his oxygen level dropped to about 88, which is rather low. It had been low like this at home, which is probably why he was sleeping so much. "You are going home with oxygen, Bill, we'll see if that helps you feel better." I wasn't surprised, but I knew Bill was.

Once oxygen is ordered by a physician, the patient cannot go home or leave the hospital until there is oxygen delivered to where the patient will be going. When the nurse called the company to order the oxygen, she was told it would be several hours before it would be delivered. This meant Bill would have to stay in the hospital until I went home, received the delivery, and then returned and picked him up.

"I am not staying here, take me home, I'll be fine." He

would not stay, so I brought him home and put him to bed and waited for the delivery. It was not a good decision on his part, I believe, but when he's made up his mind, it's final. Thankfully he didn't have any problems while we waited for the delivery.

The oxygen arrived about five hours after we got home. I didn't know what to expect would be coming. Eight small oxygen tanks called an "E" tank were put in my dining room. We were to put one of them in a small metal trolley with wheels to hold it upright so Bill could walk around the house while he pulled it with him. This would not work because he could not use his walker and pull an oxygen tank along with him. I would have to trail behind him, pulling the tank everywhere he wanted to go.

These tanks only lasted about three to four hours each, so I would have to change tanks as soon as one ran out, so he had oxygen 24/7. I would get up in the middle of the night to change the tanks when they ran out because Bill could not do this for himself. It also meant that these tanks would not last but a day or two, and then we would have to have another delivery.

Bill eventually had more testing as an outpatient to try and determine why his oxygen level kept dropping. A specialized CT scan showed that Bill had Idiopathic Pulmonary Fibrosis (IPF). It is a disease that causes scarring (fibrosis) in the lungs. The word "idiopathic" means it has no known cause. Or, as I liked to call it - idiot pulmonary fibrosis because it was so dumb to get a disease with no known cause.

We had a visit with a pulmonologist to explain every-thing to us, "The scarring or fibrosis causes stiffness in the lungs and makes it difficult to breathe. Because the heart and the brain require a steady supply of oxygen to function properly, they are also affected." He paused and then continued, "There is no known cure for the disease, if you were younger, we would see if you were eligible for a lung transplant."

Bill asked, "So how long do I have, what will happen at the end?" The doctor very kindly told him, "You could have two to four years to live, maybe longer. You will get increasingly short of breath and cough more and more. I'll order some inhalers you can use to help with the coughing, and you will have to remain on oxygen for the rest of your life."

Whooooosh, it felt like the air got sucked out of the room when he finished speaking.

Neither of us had much to say at this point. We were in shock and a bit dumbfounded, not to mention grief stricken. The doctor then said, "I will order an oxygen concentrator for your home so you don't have to drag tanks around, it will be much easier for you that way." Neither of us had seen an oxygen concentrator and weren't quite sure what to expect. We were in for an education when it arrived with all the issues and concerns that came through the door with it.

I slowly pushed Bill to the car in the wheelchair. I fought back tears, thinking of what his life would be like from now on, and wondered, how long would he be with me.

An Education in Oxygen

Lesson: How Not to Blow Up the House

When we returned from the hospital after Bill was told he would need oxygen, we really weren't quite sure what to expect would be delivered. We also didn't know where it came from, who brought it and what our responsibilities would be.

After Bill went to bed, I waited patiently for the oxygen to arrive. Well, maybe not patiently, but more curious than anything. About six hours later, a huge truck parked in front of the house with what looked like about fifty oxygen tanks in the back of it. My first thought; I hope the driver is never in an accident, or all those oxygen tanks would explode and cause a huge fire. What a dumb thing to think at this point!

The driver brought in the eight "E" tanks I talked about previously with a metal holder that looked like a milk bottle holder from years ago. This would secure the tanks, so they didn't fall or get knocked over. I had him put them in the dining room, sort of out of the way, but not really. You can't put that many tanks in a room without them being in the way. It took up a lot of space, and we would have to learn to maneuver around them. Even the dog looked at them like they were strange, but she never bothered them or seemed to care about them.

I was shown how to operate the tanks, check the pressure, and set up the regulator, as it is called for each tank. Regulators seem to be precious items, probably expensive, as they only left one that I would have to move from tank to tank when one ran out of oxygen, and I had to switch to another. Bill could not do this, so I was totally in charge of the equipment.

I signed all the paperwork and asked, "Where do you bring the tanks from, where is the warehouse?" "It's about an hour away depending on traffic, so you always want to call as soon as you need more tanks." I told him, "Well, I might as well order now because if each tank only lasts about three hours, we are going to run out soon." "I have a larger tank to bring in that you should use in an emergency, like a power failure or if we can't get here in time."

He went back out to the truck and brings a HUGE tank, almost as big as me, called an "M" tank. He also told me, "They are called oxygen cylinders, not tanks, so when you call that's what you need to tell them you need."

He used a big wrench to attach the regulator. I was a little worried I would have to do the same thing, but he said, "You only have to turn it on with this handle now." He hands me this little plastic handle with a hole in it that fits the top of the regulator. "Don't lose it!" He handed me the paperwork and left.

The regulator is what you set the number of liters of oxygen required by the patient. Oxygen is delivered in liters. The oxygen was delivered to Bill through what is called a nasal cannula, clear tubing that attached to the source of the oxygen and then goes around the ears with two small prongs that sit in the nose.

Bill was to be on two liters per minute. I had set many regulators when I worked in the hospital, and I had a respiratory therapist explain to me many times what "liters per minute" meant. "Think of it as a medication with all the same rules, like never running out and giving it on time in the right amount."

Liter flow is the amount of oxygen you receive from the cylinder of oxygen or in a hospital from the wall device that is set up. Every liter of oxygen increases the percentage of oxygen provided by about 3 to 4 percent. It is not 100 percent oxygen as the person is also breathing room air at the same time, which dilutes it.

This is technical, but I think it's interesting and clears up some confusion about a person receiving oxygen.

- The oxygen flow rate is the number set on the oxygen flow meter or on the regulator, usually between one and fifteen liters per minute. The average is about two liters per minute, depending on the patient's condition and need for oxygen.

- FiO2, which you really won't deal with at home, but respiratory therapists do when a patient is on a ventilator. For the average oxygen user, it means the percentage or concentration of oxygen that a person inhales. Room air, as we call the air we breathe normally, is made up of about 21% oxygen, 78% nitrogen, and 1% trace minerals.

What this all means is that if a person is on two liters of oxygen per minute, they are getting about 28 percent more oxygen or an FiO2 of 28 percent. This is complicated, but my point is the only way to get 100 percent oxygen is for the patient to have a breathing tube down into their lungs with 100 percent oxygen flowing through it. FiO2 is pronounced – F-eye-oh-two.

I was constantly nagging Bill to keep his oxygen on once he started wearing it. He'd leave it in the chair or take it off when he went to the bathroom. Or just take it off because he was tired of wearing it. I had to remind myself that he was only increasing his oxygen by 28 percent when it was set at two liters per minute, so taking it off for a while did not drop his oxygen level that fast or that much if he didn't leave it off for a long time. Instead of my telling Bill to breathe, I would try to instead and quit nagging him.

His pulmonologist told me to adjust the oxygen liter flow higher as needed if Bill's PO2 dropped below ninety-two. We checked it often with a little handheld device, and I have only had to raise the liters per minute to four or five a few times.

The basic oxygen rules for keeping everyone safe include:

- Place a sign on your door or to the entrance to your home that says oxygen is in use.
- No smoking by anyone in the home.
- Stay six feet away from a flame, like a gas stove.
- Avoid using flammable liquids near the source of the oxygen.
- If you leave the house with oxygen, stay at least six feet away from a flame, spark, or fire, especially in a restaurant.

The hardest rule for Bill was staying away from the gas stove. He was the cook of the family, and this would require some major changes for him. It worked out because he also didn't feel very well, so didn't want to cook anyway.

We had frequent oxygen deliveries until we saw the pulmonologist that ordered the oxygen concentrator for the house. This machine didn't take up as much room as the oxygen cylinders, but it was a little noisy. It is on every day, all day, unless we leave the house. It's mechanical sounding and makes a sound like a deep inhale, and then a burst of an exhale. We have had one for almost three years now. I still hear it in the background all the time. It, too, was placed in the dining room, which helps at night because we don't hear it in the bedroom.

The concentrator also had a longer tubing to supply the oxygen to Bill. The small tanks just used the nasal cannula tubing, which is about six feet long to supply the oxygen. So, the tanks had to move when Bill did. The concentrator could force enough oxygen through a much longer tubing. Fifty feet, in fact! This tubing is green and allowed Bill to access almost all of the house.

We got used to it quickly, and I could always find Bill by following the green tubing since it was usually attached to him. Sometimes he would get his feet wrapped in it and almost trip, or he would lasso the dog. The dog would just stand up and untangle herself, and walk away. Generally, it worked fine, and we didn't have a lot of trouble with it. This tubing is changed every month, and the cannula tubing is changed every two weeks. Both get cleaned daily.

There is a small water bottle attached to the concentrator that humidifies the oxygen before it gets to Bill to prevent the nasal passages of his nose from drying out. The water bottle needed to have the distilled water replaced in it about every eight hours, and it and the filters on the machine had to be cleaned twice a week in a vinegar solution.

An oxygen concentrator is a machine about two feet tall and a foot and a half wide by one foot thick. It must plug into a wall socket, not shared by any other device, and sit about six inches from the wall. What this machine does is concentrate the oxygen out of room air. It selectively removes the nitrogen from the air and then supplies only oxygen out the flowmeter. It's a marvelous device, and it means oxygen cylinders or tanks are no longer needed. All but one, that is, the giant cylinder remains by the concentrator's side, just in case of an emergency like a power failure.

The only problem with having the large oxygen concentrator is that we had no small cylinders that we could take in the car if we had to go somewhere. There are small concentrators available that are quite expensive, and fortunately, Bill's insurance covered the cost of rental for him. In fact, all the equipment is rented and maintained by the distributor for our insurance company.

I drove Bill to the company that supplied these small concentrators after the doctor ordered it to see if he could pass the test to use one. I said a silent prayer that he would, or he would never get out of the house. They advertise these machines on television, and they look light weight and easy to carry, about the size of a woman's purse. On TV, the person carrying one doesn't look like they even need oxygen and walks unaided and looks healthy.

In reality, the machines are heavy and a bit unwieldy

because of their size and weight. Bill could not carry it and use his walker at the same time. There is also a vent that cannot be blocked, or the machine shuts off because it overheats. The battery only lasts about two to four hours, depending on the liter flow, so it must be charged every time it is used.

There is a difference between the portable concentrator and the large one at home that is rather significant, as well. The small concentrator only puts out a puff of oxygen when the wearer takes a breath. The large concentrator constantly pours out oxygen, no matter what the person is doing. Bill had to be able to tolerate the small puff of air without his P02 dropping for him to be able to use one. Thankfully he did fine, and we brought the little gem home with us.

On the way home, Bill said, "Finally, some freedom!" It was true it did give him a new outlook that he would be able to get out of the house occasionally. It was one more thing to carry, but I was not complaining. This would allow us to leave the house together for an errand and perhaps a lunch at a restaurant.

I would often tell Bill that getting him ready to go in the car was like packing for a baby with all his mobility devices, oxygen, urinal and throw-up bags. He would nod and say, "Take your time, I'll wait until you are ready." Never acknowledging all the equipment he needed because it was just the way things were now. It also wouldn't do any good to complain about it. This was our life, and we were happy to be living it the way it was.

I Was Not Put on This Earth to Grocery Shop and Cook

Lesson: Ordering Groceries Online

As Bill was beginning to have more and more trouble walking and standing, cooking was getting harder for him. He had always been the "chief cook and bottle washer" in our home, and I loved it. He and his mother spent many hours cooking together, and he was an expert at creating wonderful dinners, whether they were simple or complicated. He had also been to cooking school in San Francisco several years earlier and enjoyed collecting recipe books and experimenting with new culinary creations.

The end of his cooking came when he had to start using oxygen. Our stove was gas, and he had to stay six feet away from a fire, pilot light, or anything hot with oxygen running through plastic tubing into his nose. Following this new rule would be hard for Bill because he loved cooking so much. I took over to make it easier for him, but I kept him involved as much as possible by having him give me cooking directions or he would look for recipes while he read the paper. Eventually, he gave up cooking completely and left it to me.

Bill also loved doing the grocery shopping to get the items for his recipes. He could no longer do this unless I took him to the store and got him an electric cart because he could no longer walk around the store. To be truthful, this fun part of his life was disappearing, and it was up to me to fill in and keep him as active as possible.

I never learned to cook much, my mother was a horrible cook, and when I worked at the hospital, I ate dinner there. I had to learn this new task quickly, or we would be eating take-out for the rest of our lives. Once in a while was okay, but not all the time. If we ordered take-out food, I would pick it up at the restaurant unless they delivered, which was like having a night off.

I started out with simple items like pasta, soups, frozen pizzas, steak and potatoes, salads, hot dogs (Bill's favorite), hamburgers, and fries. Microwaved frozen dinners were okay occasionally, but I didn't think we should eat all the sodium that is in those meals. They were not a great choice to help someone get stronger and stay nourished.

One Christmas, we had a frozen turkey in the freezer, and I told Bill, "I'm going to cook this thing, doesn't seem like it's too hard to cook a turkey." I thawed it out, rubbed some butter on it, and shoved it in the oven. I did put it in a cooking pan first. He helped me make the dressing he loved, and that would go in the oven later. I could manage mashed potatoes and vegetables, so I felt we were set for our Christmas dinner. If it turned out bad, we'd eat all the side dishes with cranberry sauce, and it would just go down as a bad attempt at cooking a turkey.

It smelled delicious, and my hopes were up for a great meal. I took the turkey out of the oven, we sampled it, and it was fabulous. I made gravy, don't ask me how I knew how, but I've always known how to make gravy. We sat down to dinner. I looked at our plates of food and said, "Oops, I forgot to cook the dressing. Guess we will have it tomorrow." My dinner turned out delicious even without the dressing, but then Bill said, "If you can cook a turkey dinner, you can cook anything, so I'll let you do it all now!" Guess I did too good of a job.

I'll admit, I was spoiled, and this cooking idea was more than I expected it to be. It was work trying to come up with ideas! Planning food and buying it with the thoughts of a dinner another day later in the week was starting to keep me running in circles. I asked myself many times, "How do mothers with children, who might also work, do this every day?" I had a new respect for anyone who thinks up and cooks dinner, not to mention lunch and some breakfast every day.

My recipes would become more elaborate, and I sounded like I knew what I was doing a lot of the time, but not always. When Bill was doing the cooking, about 11:00 a.m. every day, sometimes earlier, I would ask, "What's for dinner?" This always made him laugh, and he would say, "What do you want?" We would plan the meal together then. Now all of this had gotten turned around, and he asked me, "What's for dinner?" and I asked him, "What do you want?"

When the cooking and shopping got added to my list of duties, I really felt I was in over my head. I knew we wouldn't starve, but I also knew I had a lot to learn. I tried not to let it consume me, and when Bill wanted to help, I would let him, even if it was just chopping onions. I never really learned to love cooking as some people do, but I managed.

As time went on, I got better at planning and cooking, but there were days I would be tired or not feeling well, and I would say, "I'm not cooking, what can I order for dinner?" Bill would laugh, and we would come up with something, even if it were bacon and eggs or waffles for dinner. Those were both our favorite meals for dinner, so it was not a problem. Bill also would eat a meatloaf sandwich or soup or something small without a complaint. Mind you, the meatloaf was purchased at the store, I didn't make it.

Bill used to always say when he had a good meal, either in a restaurant or at someone's home, "It was terrible, just terrible." He was kidding, of course, and most people laughed. I asked him to quit saying it because I was just too sensitive with my new task of cooking and might believe him. He kindly stopped saying "terrible" and now says, "It was just perfect, thank you." I couldn't ask for more. If only cooking the groceries was as easy as picking them up!

With all the cooking came all the grocery shopping. I used to shop with Bill when he could walk and get around the store, and he would have the list memorized. I had to carry the list with a pen to cross off the items, or I spent more time looking at the list than shopping. I also only bought what was on the list with an occasional "impulse" buy of something that looked good in the fruit or the muffins and cookie departments. I was getting pretty good about shopping, frequenting the three main grocery stores in the area.

In 2020, the pandemic hit, and shopping was almost forbidden as we went into a lockdown that March. I discovered shopping online and picking up the groceries the next day. What an invention, and so easy. This became my new way of shopping for just about everything. I could order one day, choose my pick-up time, drive to the store at that time the next day, and the groceries would be put in my car by the nice people who worked for the store. I could be back home in thirty minutes. Bill was fine for that length of time by himself.

I was amazed at how great a job the store clerks did in filling my grocery orders for this free service. Vegetables were nice, the fruit was always fresh, and the meat and laundry products were kept separate in plastic bags. Occasionally there was a substitution if they were out of a product, but not often. I learned the best days to order, which were generally Tuesday and Wednesday, and not to put in three pounds when I was really trying to get three bananas.

I would soon learn to work with online shopping and an occasional trip to the store with Bill so he could shop for the items he loved, like cream puffs and mortadella, which I didn't buy. It got easier as time went on, but I never really thought of myself as a great cook or a terrific shopper. I was so lucky that Bill would accept what I put in front of him and eat it with a smile on his face.

Bill's Idea of Grocery Shopping

Lesson: Humor - Don't Leave it at Home

On Sunday of Memorial Day weekend, I was going to the small Walmart in our town that carries a lot of interesting things to eat that the larger grocery stores don't carry. Indian Simmer Sauces and Mexican food and condiments, as well as great vegetables. I got dressed, and was finding my purse, and asked Bill, "Do you want to go with me, so you can browse around? He said, "Sure, let me get ready."

We were in his SUV with all our shopping bags and the list in just a short time. His small oxygen concentrator was plugged in and set for the five liters of oxygen he was using at the time. The store wasn't very far away, so it would be an easy trip, and he could see what was happening downtown and the surrounding area where we lived.

We passed a new home building site on our way, and they had just opened the model homes, so I said, "Let's go check it out for a minute, I'll just drive in and come back out." "Sure," he said, so I went straight through the signal instead of turning left, where I would normally go. The entrance was beautiful but not finished yet. We could see the model homes and the new lodge they were building that would house the gym and offices for the administration. There would eventually be a pool, as well as tennis and pickleball courts and a dog park.

I turned around in their parking lot as the streets were blocked off, so I couldn't drive any further and came back out and went toward the grocery store. It was just a little detour. But it made the trip a little more interesting for Bill since he seldom got out of the house to see any new buildings or roads.

When we got to the grocery store, one of their electric carts was already outside near a handicapped parking place. I saw it as I drove in. "Look Bill, they have the cart outside for you by a great parking spot. This trip was fortuitous!" I parked, got out of the car, and walked to the electric cart, got in and drove it to his side of the car. We put the oxygen concentrator in the basket of the cart, Bill got into the seat, and we were off to the store.

Normally I would have had to park, walk into the store, find an electric cart, drive it out to Bill, help him get out of the car and get him seated in the cart and then return to the store with him driving the cart. It wasn't a big deal, but I knew that with Bill along, this trip was going to take twice as long anyway, so this was a bit of a time saver. I really don't need to be in a hurry, yet I always feel I'm in a hurry for some reason. Having the cart outside was a luxury.

When we got inside, we were on the pharmacy, dog food, and paper goods side of the store, so I told Bill, "I'm going to get Kleenex and the dog treats." I was thinking he would follow behind me, just a little slower. I was wrong and should have known better.

I walked down a few aisles, didn't hear the motor of the cart behind me, turned around, and Bill was not there. I started wandering the aisles, calling his name. "Bill, where are you?" I kept searching, no Bill anywhere near where I had told him I was going. I knew he couldn't be far, and the cart was huge, so I should have been able to spot him easily. I found the Kleenex and turned around and started back toward where I thought Bill would be, and out he popped from one of the aisles. "Where did you go?" "I was looking at the school supply stuff for the clear sticky markers for my books." We continued to shop as I walked away, wondering what he would do next.

Bill liked to go down every aisle and find things that are not on the list, I don't shop that way, but this trip was meant so Bill could do some looking around. I walked away thinking he would be behind me, turned around, and he had gone in some other direction or would be 40 feet behind me. I would then have to go find him again.

The little basket on the cart began to fill up, so my grocery bags didn't fit anymore. I took them out to carry them, and as I'm doing this, I noticed Bill's oxygen concentrator had an error message. "Low oxygen – turn off and recharge." It seemed fine, but if it truly wasn't working, we needed to get back to the car and plug it in to charge. "Don't worry about it," Bill says, "I'm fine." I walked away, shaking my head, hoping he was right.

We visited all the aisles Bill wanted to see, and then got to the produce department, which is crowded with other shoppers and a guy with a huge cart filling an online shopping order. I hate their carts; they are so big and always in the way. Bill decided he wanted to pass by the cart, said, "Excuse me," to the guy. The guy moved the cart. I asked, "What are you looking for?" "Nothing, I just wanted to look." The guy grimaced at him. I think I did too.

The oxygen concentrator was still acting funny, the error message kept popping up, so I headed to the checkout stand. I always do self-checkout, so I don't have to unload the groceries, have the clerk scan them, bag them, and then load them back in the cart again. I took each item out of the cart, scanned it, and then placed it back in the cart to be bagged later. It goes very fast and no one else handles the groceries.

Our vehicle was in the first parking spot out the door. I walked there, opened the trunk so I could put the heavy items in before helping Bill get back in the car. Bill followed close behind me and stopped behind the back of the car so I could finish loading the groceries into the trunk. When he tried to move the cart to the passenger side of the car so he could get out, it wouldn't start up again. The battery was dead!

I told him, "Sit tight, I'll go get somebody in the store to help." I unloaded the rest of the groceries, and while I'm doing this the oxygen concentrator began alarming again. I thought to myself, "Errrrr, damn… why did I think this cart was a good idea when it had not been charged?" Yet one more lesson.

I ran inside and found a clerk standing by the door and told him, "We have one of your electric carts and the battery has gone dead. It's sitting right behind my car, so I can't back up." He yelled over to another clerk, "Hey, Marco, we need to carry an electric cart in!" Marco replied, "Oh no! Okay, I'll be right there."

As we headed out the door, I said, "But the first thing we have to do is get my husband out of it!" They could see Bill was still in the cart. I noticed some hesitation on their part, so I said, "It's okay, I can get him out." I thought to myself, "Please be able to stand and walk a few feet."

I helped Bill out of the cart, and he hung onto the car to walk to the passenger side. While I helped Bill one of the men sat in the cart and got it to run for a bit, so it didn't have to be carried into the store. What a relief. I plugged in Bill's oxygen concentrator and crossed my fingers it would be okay for the trip home.

As I drove home, I thought about the shopping adventure we just had. It now seemed comical when I thought of what we must have looked like in the store. Me, searching for Bill, "Bill, where are you? And Bill looking happy as a clam and not paying one bit of attention to me as he wandered around.

I had a little conversation with myself on the drive home. "Calm down, Bill's fine, we didn't have to call for an ambulance, and he had a good time." I then started to laugh because this would have made a fabulous, humorous YouTube video if anyone had been watching us try and get around the store and then have the cart die in the parking lot. I would try and remember the humor in it and remind myself to take my good humor with me when we went anywhere.

When we got home, I unpacked the groceries, and Bill went to bed. He was worn out and would rest for several hours. My day continued and I finished up my Sunday chores after putting the groceries away.

The trip to the store was a bit of extra work for me, but Bill enjoyed the outing, which seemed to be the more important thing, not the crazy way it happened. It would be repeated soon, I was sure.

When Bill got up from his nap, he asked, "When can we go to Raley's, I'm still looking for chili peppers?" I rolled my eyes privately and said, "Just give me a day or two to recover from today's adventure and we can go."

He was happy with that answer, and I knew we would be back in the car soon, so he could look for the chili peppers he was determined to purchase. He had a recipe in his pocket he wanted me to make. I hoped it would be a little easier and with less drama, but I never could predict these events and just had to learn to "roll with the shopping cart."

Within a few days, we were at Raley's, looking for the chili peppers Bill wanted. I went in and got him an electric cart that had been plugged in so we knew he wouldn't run out of power. Off we went shopping for what was on the list and all the goodies he could find that were not on the list. One specialty at this store was meatloaf! Bill loved it, and it was one of the first things he put in the shopping cart.

This was a much quieter shopping trip, no drama, not as much laughter, but it was done, and we could move on to the next shopping adventure, which I would make alone, or order online until Bill felt like going with me again. He was often too tired to go shopping with me, but he did enjoy it when he could. We told the story of the dead electric cart in the Walmart parking lot several times, and it always made us laugh. This laughter made the whole trip worthwhile.

Hiring and Firing Help

Lesson: You Are the Expert

About a year after Bill was diagnosed with IPF (Idiopathic pulmonary fibrosis) and my lupus and rheumatoid arthritis were making it more difficult for me to keep up with things, we decided to get some help a couple of days a week. Bill had paid into a long-term care policy for years, and we thought it was time to start using the benefits of the policy. Sounds easy enough, but it's a bit of a long and winding road to get it all approved and put into action.

The first thing we did was call the long-term care company to find out what the whole process would be and what we needed to do at our end. This turned into a forty-five-minute call, as the man who answered our questions would also be filing a claim for us. After Bill answered several questions about his health issues and medications, he was asked why he needed help. What were his physical limitations that he thought qualified him for help? We did not know that there must be difficulty with at least three activities of daily living (ADLs) that the company considers necessary for you to file a claim.

Bill told him he needed help walking and used a walker;

he no longer drove and could no longer cook because of his oxygen use 24/7. The representative asked several more questions about dressing himself and toileting, as well as some simple questions to test his cognitive ability. Bill was getting very tired, so he gave very brief answers to the questions. The representative said the claim would go to a nurse, and we would get a phone call with more questions, and an assessment of Bill's health would be done. This was during the Covid lockdown, so it would have to be done by phone when normally there would have been a nurse coming to the house.

It was interesting to us that Bill paid for his policy in California, but it was administered from Minnesota. Soon a call from Minnesota came, and another lengthy conversation ensued. After about an hour, Bill again was exhausted. This was when the nurse decided to ask the questions to determine cognitive decline. He did not do well, and the nurse told him someone would be in touch again with more questions. Bill groaned; these were long hard phone calls for him.

We were mailed some information that told us there are six activities of daily living that are used to determine the need for long-term care. The ADLs include mobility, bathing, feeding, using the restroom unaided, dressing, and regulating/taking medications. If the individual can't do three out of the six ADLs, they could qualify for long-term care. Help with eating made sense, but not qualifying because you can't cook for yourself did not.

We received three more phone calls and finally got the determination that Bill could have 24/7 help. This was more than we had planned on, but if anything happened to me, it would be useful so I could get him care at night too. We had to pay for ninety days of service out of pocket first, and then the long-term care insurance would begin to pay. We needed to find a caregiver quickly and start paying before the policy could go into effect.

I had begun searching for help while we were still answering questions and talking to the long-term care company waiting for final approval. We lived in a retirement community with many health care providers in the area so thought it would be easy to find some help. After all, we are all getting older and eventually would need some type of assistance, whether it be at home or in a facility. It wasn't hard to find companies, what was difficult was the interview process that was very tedious for Bill.

Each company would send a representative to assess him, asking the same questions as the previous company. He would ask me, "Do I have to keep answering the same questions over and over?" I had to nod and say, "Yes, I'm afraid that's how it works."

I would show them the house and what we had done to make things easier for Bill. Grab bars were near all toilets and the showers, a cane was at every doorway, and we had two walkers. The wheelchairs and scooter were in the garage.

We easily found a local company that Bill liked, and we felt comfortable with. Within a week, we had a caregiver come to the house, along with the manager of our account to meet us. She was a lovely young woman, and we thought it was a perfect match. We had to have her a minimum of four hours a day, so we chose Monday and Friday from 9:00 a.m. to 1:00 p.m.

At first, I wasn't exactly sure what she would do for four hours. Bill often slept most of that time, and because she was hired for him, the work had to be related to him. But soon, we determined that cleaning, laundry, dishes, changing the bed, and cooking were the jobs that she, as a non-medical care worker, could do. There was plenty to keep her busy.

I slowly introduced her to our needs for cleaning and laundry and some cooking, and we thought we were set. She lasted two weeks. It was troubling. We enjoyed her company, and she was such a nice woman I really didn't want her to go. I spent so much time training her I didn't know if I had the energy to do it again for someone else. We wondered, "What had we done to make her quit?"

She sent us a lovely card, "I'm sorry I can't work for you anymore, my mother is ill, and I need to take care of her." We felt very bad for her, but we understood her need to take care of family first, but we would now have to find someone else, and I wasn't looking forward to it.

Within a week, the company had found someone new and brought her over. I'll admit I wasn't very nice when I said, "If you think this isn't going to work out for you, please don't take the job, I can't keep going through this." She responded, "I have no intention of quitting." I was concerned she wouldn't last because she drove over 45 minutes to get to us. I thought she would get tired of the drive. I found out later Chrissy would only drive back roads and avoided the highway, which made her trip even longer.

We had other concerns as we got to know her that she had a lot going on in her life. She was very petite, and amazing to us - sixty years old. She was a hard worker but tended to have injuries that prevented her from doing things like vacuuming. She took care of her husband at home, who was in a wheelchair, and had two adult special needs children that also kept her very busy. We loved her immediately, and that included our dog, who would hear her drive up and go crazy barking until she got to the door.

We added some more hours to her schedule and had created a nice routine. I didn't have to repeat directions for what I wanted to be done; she would just do the jobs on her own. I could leave her a note if I were going to be gone, giving her the chores for the day. She never complained. She helped Bill shower and get dressed and took care of making the bed, as I could no longer pull on a fitted sheet because my hands hurt so much from arthritis. She was a great cook as well. I would give her the dinner recipe, and she would prepare it after she had done all her other chores. My house has never been so clean!

Chrissy would sometimes need to take some time off to take care of her husband, and her manager at the care company would call and ask if we wanted a replacement. We accepted a replacement one time for a couple of days. She was a lovely woman too, and really took good care of Bill, but Chrissy returned very soon after that. When they would call again and tell me, "Chrissy needs to take a few days off, do you want a replacement?" I would say, "No, we are fine, we'll wait for Chrissy." I don't think I could give a better recommendation than that.

Since I was nervous about leaving Bill alone, Chrissy being at the house gave me a couple of hours to run errands, get groceries, or go to the doctor. It was a relief to know that if something happened to Bill, that she would get a hold of me immediately. I never went far away, so she knew I would get home as soon as possible if I were needed.

Many days she and I worked together on a project. We cleaned the kitchen shelves, and rearranged all the dishes, and pots and pans, as well as cleaned the closets. Bill began packing up books to give to the library, and Chrissy would put them in the car for me since lifting was becoming difficult for me. I began to rely on her more and more. I thought she liked coming to help us as much as we liked having her with us. I think we were incredibly lucky to get her with the first company we hired.

After ninety days, Bill's long-term care kicked in, and Chrissy's company did all the billing for us. When Chrissy would arrive and leave, she would have to check in and out on her cell phone to let the company know when she arrived and what she had done for Bill each time she was here. It seemed like a very simple system, but I saw her have difficulty with it occasionally and hoped it wasn't too much trouble for her. We gave her enough to do so she didn't need to struggle with getting her hours documented so she could get paid.

Six months after Bill's long-term care was being paid for out of his account, he got a phone call from a nurse administrator at the company asking how he was doing. A five-minute conversation led to a reduction in the hours they would pay for. Four hours a day, seven days a week was the new ruling. This made no sense; we weren't using all the hours that they had approved in the first place, and Bill's memory was getting so poor that it was unfair to talk to him for such a brief time and then make this decision.

We got a letter stating I could contest the decision by filling out a form they sent and sending it back with a copy of his medical records. I went into full, "I'll get this fixed," mode, and within five days I sent them the information from his last doctor visit, which gave evidence of his cognitive decline and documentation of his medications. I asked for a nurse to come to the house for an evaluation to get the decision changed.

We received a letter a couple of weeks later that told us a Home Health Nurse would come to visit as soon as possible to reassess Bill's need for more hours than they were allowing him with their new decision. What the forms and phone calls did not reveal to them was my illness and how it was affecting my care of him when no one else was here to help. Her visit would hopefully clear up the "picture" of his needs as well as what I wasn't able to do for him anymore.

A month later, we got a call from the nurse stating she would be coming to the house to evaluate Bill. She told me on the phone, "I live about two hours away, so please be sure you are both available and have his medication and doctor's records available." I told her, "Sure, no problem, I already have everything ready."

Kathy arrived and immediately assessed the situation. She interviewed Bill, who once again got very tired and couldn't answer all the cognitive assessment questions she asked. She toured the house and gave me some more ideas to assist him. The best suggestion was a commode by the bed, so he didn't get up to go to the bathroom at night because he was a potential fall risk.

She asked me about my medical problems as well, and after about two hours, told me, "They are wrong in reducing his hours, he needs 24/7 care, and I will tell them that."

Hallelujah, I had made some progress, and things were going to go back to "normal" for us. On her way out the door, she said, "You look awful, you need a break! Go to a hotel for a day or two or a spa." Oh, wouldn't that have been nice?

Within two weeks, I received a call from a new nurse administrator assigned to Bill at the long-term care company to tell me they were having a meeting about Bill that afternoon, and she was sure it had been a mistake to reduce his hours. "Thanks, I appreciate the call and your time." She said, "I'll talk to you tomorrow because of the 2-hour time change unless the meeting goes very quickly, then I can get back to you today."

The next day, she called, "Your hours should have never been cut, I'm sorry for the inconvenience, but we will reimburse you for the hours you paid for and institute the change immediately." I couldn't thank her enough.

The difficult issue with long-term care is you think you've paid into it, and it's your money you invested, so you should be able to use it when "you" think you need it. It is not that way; you need to make sure you understand when it can be used and how to use it. It's a long process, and many days, I would get frustrated and want to hang up the phone before I went crazy with the person on the other end when their rules didn't make sense.

Documentation is necessary for all these insurance services. Be sure you hang on to every piece of paper and letter and be able to access your loved one's medical records. But more importantly, know what you are buying in the first place and be sure it fits your needs or what you think you need or will need. And finally, don't be afraid to question the system. You are the one doing the caregiving and the paperwork. You are the expert! You know what your loved one needs and how it should happen. Even if you aren't a nurse, you know more about what is going on than the insurance companies do because you live it every day.

Eventually, we had to let Chrissy go. She was too distracted and made a few potentially dangerous mistakes. One being she left the gas burner on the stove lit after cooking Bill his lunch. Thirty minutes later, I walked into the kitchen and found it burning. The oxygen tanks were in the room next to the kitchen, ten feet away. The house could have blown up.

It was a hard decision, but leaving Bill with someone I was more worried about than him just didn't make sense. We had to begin a search for a new caregiver. We were told by several people at the insurance company it was better to hire a caregiver before you think you need one. Since you must pay for ninety days out of pocket anyway even if you have long-term care insurance. If you wait too long, you might have trouble finding one, and you will wear yourself out doing all the care yourself.

Here are some resources for locating caregiver services that I referred to:

Family Caregiver Alliance
National Center on Caregiving
(800) 445-8106
Website: www.Caregiver.org
Email: info@caregiver.org

Government Services
Administration for Community Living
www.ACL.gov
Benefits Check-Up
Designed by the National Council on Aging, this website enables you to complete a questionnaire to find federal, state, and local programs that you might be eligible for and how to apply.
www. BenefitsCheckup.org

Eldercare Locator
The Eldercare Locator helps older adults and their caregivers find local services, including health insurance counseling, free and low-cost legal services, and contact information for Area Agencies on Aging. (AAA).
Eldercare.acl.gov

Well Spouse Association
www.WellSpouse.org

Aging Life Care Association
www.AgingLifeCare.org

National Academy of Elder Law Attorney
www.NAELA.org

Other good places to start to look for help for your loved one or yourself are senior centers, independent living centers, local agencies on aging, local chapters of national organizations, and foundations such as the Alzheimer's Association, Brain Injury Association, Multiple Sclerosis

Society, and Parkinson's groups. Community mental health centers, social services or case management agencies, and church groups may be other good sources to find assistance as well. You might find these in the phone book under "Social Services" or "Seniors."

It can be stressful having another person in the house, so to make it as easy as possible, try some of these ideas.

- Be sure you know what your caregiver is allowed to do by their agency.
- Set boundaries and standards of care by example.
- Don't ask the caregiver to do things you won't do, unless you can't do them.
- The caregiver is a guest in your home. They should act appropriately and be respectful.
- You are in charge! You know what you and your loved one need.
- Print out a list of the things you would like accomplished with each visit.

  For example:
  1. Bathing
  2. General Personal Care
  3. Bed making
  4. Laundry
  5. Cooking
  6. Housekeeping
  7. Garbage Out
  8. Blood Pressure
  9. Pulse
  10. Oxygen level

- Provide maps or advice on shortcuts to your home if it makes their travel to and from easier.

- Show them around the neighborhood if they aren't familiar with where you live, places like the grocery store or the gas station.

- Share your phone numbers and contact information and get theirs in return.

- What would you like your caregiver to wear? Scrubs are a good idea because they give a professional appearance and create a health-giving environment.

- Set rules for using the phone while working if you have a preference.

- Should they wear a mask?

- Have all cleaning products available and be sure the caregiver knows where they are.

- If you have a pet, do they need to take them for a walk or let them outside? Are there rules about treats for your pet or feeding them?

- The caregiver is there to help your loved one, not family members who may think they are there to get them coffee and serve lunch.

These are just a few examples; every case is different. Go slow, and you will discover what works best for you and your loved one if you just give it some time.

Loneliness

Lesson: You Are the Master of Your Own Fate

While common definitions of loneliness describe it as a state of solitude, characterized by the feeling of being alone, without company or companions. It is a state of mind causing an inability to make friends because of self-doubt and low self-esteem. Loneliness causes people to feel empty, alone, and unwanted. People who are lonely often crave human contact, but their state of mind makes it more difficult to form connections with other people.

Loneliness, according to many experts, is not necessarily about being alone. Instead, if you feel alone and isolated, then that is how loneliness plays into your state of mind. Loneliness can also be a symptom of depression.

Contributing factors to loneliness include situational variables, such as physical isolation, moving to a new location, and divorce. The death of someone significant in a person's life can also lead to feelings of loneliness.

Lonely adults get less exercise than those who are not lonely. Their diet is higher in fat, their sleep is less efficient, and they report more daytime fatigue. Loneliness also disrupts the regulation of cellular processes causing us to prematurely age. I thought I could see this happening when I looked at my face, but then again, I could have been seeing fatigue.

I had always been able to keep busy with sewing, knitting, and quilting, but there were days when nothing replaced visiting with another human being. I had many years of depression, and the constant drain of never knowing when Bill would fall ill again was difficult for me. I felt depression seeping back into my life. I had to learn to adapt or go crazy that was a simple fact.

Bill was sleeping all the time. Many days, he would get up in the morning, nap, get up for lunch, nap, get up for dinner, and then go to bed at 8:00 p.m. One Christmas, he slept until 3:00 p.m. and did not remember it was Christmas until I put the prime rib in the oven for dinner.

The house had to be kept quiet while Bill slept during the day. All my hobbies and activities were relatively quiet, and I would try to keep the dog from barking and the phone from ringing. I shut the door to the laundry room so he wouldn't hear the dryer and never went in the bedroom while he was asleep. This limited my ability to do laundry, get dressed, or clean the house.

I generally walked the dog in the morning after my breakfast depending on the weather, and then when I got home, Bill would get up, and I would fix his breakfast. Bill would go back to bed then, and if I had a bad night, I would lay down and nap with him. If he wasn't up, I didn't have to make sure he was safe, so I could rest.

Poor sleep has always been an issue for me, and it is

another sign of loneliness and depression. I was often up until 3:00 or 4:00 a.m. or took so much sleep medication I couldn't hold my eyes open during the day. I could see that this was only getting worse.

I began to look for ways to stay busy, quiet, and at home if Bill needed me, but still have some outside activities that kept me from being isolated. My biggest entertainment some days was texting my friend in Utah about ten times a day, and she would text back. We sent videos of clouds, our dogs, our flowers, or just wished each other a "good morning" and then "good night" every single day. We seldom spoke on the phone; the messages were enough.

Another activity that let someone else in the world know all was well here was to play a game on my phone called "Words with Friends." It's a scrabble game that you play with someone on another phone. I generally lost but the fact that if I didn't play a word by a certain time of day, I would get a message asking, "Are you okay?" At least I knew someone was out there that was checking on me and would call if I didn't play the game.

I also joined a group of quilters that made quilts for veterans. The group is known as Quilts of Valor. It's nationwide and presents thousands of quilts a year to our special veterans who have served so proudly in the military. When you are a quilter, you have generally made quilts for everyone you can think of, but you still want to quilt, so finding a worthy place to donate quilts was a very good way to spend time and have other quilters to talk to. I made and donated several quilts over the years, and I had done most of the quilting for the local group on my longarm quilting machine. It's a very worthy project, and I fllled many a lonely day working on quilts for this group.

I tried focusing on relationships with people with common interests who lived nearby and would perhaps enjoy going out for lunch occasionally. I've never been good at making friends and tend to do better if I stayed quiet at home, but I knew if I didn't want to spend the rest of my days completely alone, I needed to work on this a little harder.

Then I wondered, "What about Bill?" He only had me, and Chris, his friend that came by about once a month or so to visit and have a beer. Bill looked forward to these visits so much, but was that enough for him? He was lonely too, I thought, and was not any better at making friends than I was. We were quite a matched set, and loving each other would not sustain either of us when the other one passed away.

Bill took a leap one day and started contacting some of the attorneys that had worked for him before he retired. He had hired many women when he was Chief Counsel, and they adored him. He was a great mentor, understanding and compassionate both at work and home. He had several emails from some of his ex-employees and a phone call occasionally. The thing is, they weren't really "his" employees. They worked for the state too, but he did the hiring and was their boss. The state paid their salaries. I didn't know all of them, well I knew names, but not faces. When two of the women said they wanted to come to visit, I was all for it.

I made lunch, and the "two ladies," as Bill called them, brought dessert from our favorite bakery when we lived in Sacramento. In fact, this bakery had made our wedding cake. We had a great afternoon, lots of reminiscing and storytelling. Almost all the attorneys that worked for Bill are retired now but remain close to each other. I had the feeling that Bill's health issues would go out over the internet, and we would hear from more of his friends and employees.

That's exactly what happened too. Several people started checking on him, and the ladies came back about every three months and brought us lunch. He got very excited about their visits, and always had a good day when they come. He remembered he had some old pictures of birthday parties at the office he wanted to find to give them on their next visit, He found them in an old photo album, and they are sitting with some books he saved to give them on their next visit.

Of course, we could not rely on their visits and phone calls every few months to cure our "problem." We needed to take care of ourselves and our loneliness. Bill seemed to be happy with the way things were, but I would need to continue to work on this for the rest of my life. Happily, I can say that my niece, who I had not spoken to in many years, got in touch with me. Her daughter, my great-niece, got married recently. I was invited to the wedding in Texas, but I couldn't go, but I did get to hear all the details by text and email.

I've heard the saying, "old friends, are the best friends." There is a sense of security that comes with old friends. They might be able to finish your sentence for you and probably know all your quirks because they have known you so long. They can also become an extension of your family or actually your family. Hang on to your friends, and if you make new ones, be sure they stay in your life long enough to become an "old" friend.

The one thing that is important to remember is that you are the master of your own fate when it comes to loneliness. If you are feeling lonely, then maybe it's time for a change. Something is wrong, whether it be with you or your circumstances. Change is hard, go slow, and be gentle with yourself.

Every Afternoon at Three

Lesson: Find a Little Enjoyment Every Day

Bill has always enjoyed a cocktail or two before dinner. I learned to enjoy one with him, and our favorite drink was easily gin and tonic. You didn't need to be a trained bartender to fix it because the ingredients were simple. During one of Bill's hospital stays, he was told he should not drink anymore. This would be a challenge, alcohol did not mix with his medications, and yet he would miss having a drink more than anyone anticipated or realized, especially me.

I didn't give much thought to how difficult it was to stop drinking, even if you only had one drink a day. When he came home from the hospital, I got rid of all the liquor and told him, "If you can't drink, then I won't either." I would have a drink if we went out to dinner, and he would stick to water or tonic with lime. It seemed simple enough, but it was not simple. It was very hard.

Sometimes Bill couldn't get to sleep. This was early on, before his IPF diagnosis and using oxygen. He would often want a brandy before bed. I kept some in the cupboard, and he would find it and fix himself a small drink. I didn't say anything but realized the brandy was disappearing rather quickly. These were not small drinks he was having.

One night, I heard a "thud" in the kitchen about midnight. He had fallen or slipped from his chair to the floor. I ran to the kitchen and tried to help him up, but I just couldn't get him off the floor because he was so heavy, not to mention a little drunk. I did not want to call for emergency help, so I came up with the idea that if he backed himself to the chair, he could sort of scoot himself up while holding on to the chair with my help. This worked, and he was upright again.

After I went back to bed I heard another "thud." He'd fallen again. I realized he probably had more to drink than I thought he had. We went through the same process and got him off the floor, but this time I got the wheelchair and pushed him to the bedroom and put him back in bed. I couldn't risk another fall.

After he woke up the next day, I asked, "Can we talk about last night?" "Oh, I'm sorry, I know I shouldn't have had all that brandy, but I just couldn't sleep." I said, "Okay, so now we have to find another way for you to get to sleep, and I am getting rid of the brandy." I had to put an end to this, or it was going to wreak havoc with his medications. I told him, "There can be no more alcohol in the house because it isn't safe for you to drink. "He looked like a contrite 5-year-old who ate too many cookies and got caught, but he agreed with me. I poured all the alcohol down the drain.

"What do you mean it isn't safe?" he then asked me, a

little angry after I poured all the liquor out. "Well, you could fall and hurt yourself if you don't pay attention to how much you are drinking, and I don't want to risk it with the side effects from your medications." He agreed, but I knew the issue was not resolved yet.

We survived quite nicely with our new "no alcohol" routine. I missed it too, but I thought it was only fair to keep alcohol out of the house if I was going to make him abide by the new rule of "no alcohol." I would substitute lemonade, iced tea, or tonic with lime if he wanted a drink in the afternoon. We were not soda drinkers, so Coke or Pepsi just wouldn't work for us. We lived on a golf course, and "Arnold Palmers" were popular here, so I started making them as well. They are a mix of iced tea and lemonade. Very refreshing.

After Bill was eventually given his terminal diagnosis after several hospital stays, I thought to myself, "If having a drink before dinner is such a simple pleasure for him, maybe I could make it work somehow." He was losing so many things in his life that maybe he could enjoy a cocktail occasionally. I thought about it for a while and decided I would buy a small bottle of gin and some tonic. But I would hide it and always be in control of it.

We had a large sitting area at the end of our kitchen with a large window that looked out toward the street. Bill read the newspaper, or his books sitting in his favorite chair there. We spent many happy hours talking or just sitting together quietly near this window.

The dog would join us in what we called "window dog position." I would pick her up and put her on the couch, and she would lean over the arm of the chair so she could stare out the window and watch the world go by. We didn't live on a very busy street, but evidently, this was entertaining enough for her.

It seemed we gathered in this manner about 3:00 p.m. everyday. We discussed our day, the news, and Bill would sometimes tell me about the books he was reading or the newspaper articles he enjoyed.

One day, I decided to surprise Bill with a small gin and tonic. It was an experiment to see if this one drink would make him as happy as I thought it would and if he could stop after just one. The alcohol was hidden in a bedroom closet, so I took a couple of small glasses and a shot glass into the bedroom, measured the alcohol into each glass, came back to the kitchen, added ice, and opened a bottle of tonic. He watched me but didn't say anything. I handed him his drink and said, "Enjoy!" Nothing more needed to be said.

This would soon become our ritual, and every day at 3:00 p.m., we would sit in the kitchen, and I would make us a drink. He probably knew where the alcohol was if he really wanted to find it, but he never tried. He knew I was trying to give him something to look forward to, something as simple as a gin and tonic in the afternoon to keep his life as normal as I could for the time being. We both enjoyed our little drink in the afternoon, and it made our time sitting together and visiting even more special.

Often, I would start preparing dinner at about 4:00 p.m. as Bill liked to eat around 5:00 p.m., and he would continue to sip his drink and offer help with the cooking if I needed it. Mostly chopping onions or getting things out of the refrigerator. His back would begin to hurt, so he couldn't stand for long, but it was almost like the old days when we fixed dinner together. Even if it was just for a few minutes, it felt like nothing had changed, and illness had not entered our home.

The only wonderful interruption to this routine was that we occasionally had a friend of Bill's that would stop by after work for a beer. Chris and Bill talked about war, history, and books. They were like father and son. Great friends and companions. Chris drank beer, so on the days he was coming, I would have beer for him, and Bill and I would split one. Sierra Nevada Pale Ale was Chris's favorite. We didn't normally drink beer, but we loved Chris so much that we would drink one with him to pass the time in congenial conversation and laughter. It was a small concession for a good friend.

I don't think Chris knew of our routine at 3:00 p.m., but he was always welcome and a very enjoyable person to have visit. Every time he left, I would walk him to the door, and he would say, "Call me if you need anything, I'm only ten minutes away." I knew he would come if I ever had to call.

This one simple pleasure made years of memories for us. It was our gathering time, our quiet time of the day. I would sometimes think I should be doing something else; I don't know what. Maybe keeping up with the housework or the garden, but I knew this time would never come again, and it was precious. No television, no interruptions, just two people who loved each other hanging on to every moment they could gather before one of them was no longer there.

My Brother has Lung Cancer

Lesson: Saying "Good-bye"

While Bill was going through his medical issues, my brother was diagnosed with lung cancer. He is my only living relative on the planet, and I was not only mad about it but grieving for him. My dad and my oldest brother both died of lung cancer as well, and it seemed to be the Wiseman's disease. They all smoked, of course, but still, it is an overwhelming diagnosis.

Charlie was given a round of radiation, and things seemed to be okay for him for a while. He also had COPD and was beginning to cough a lot because of it and would eventually need to go on oxygen. When I visited him about four years before this, he was showing signs of shortness of breath just walking through a grocery store.

He gave up his beloved golf game because he couldn't breathe and made a move from Arizona to Missouri, which was closer to his wife's children. A smart decision for them both as they would see the grandchildren more often instead of traveling to see them across several states for every holiday.

In May, I got a text message from Charlie telling me he was in the hospital with difficulty breathing. I offered as much support as possible by text but decided to call instead. He was doing okay, but it seemed the cancer had grown significantly since March. About three months. It was devastating news, and the doctors were debating what to do to reduce the tumor size so he could breathe easier.

He was in the hospital a few days, discharged, and then back again for a lung biopsy. That was done, and it was determined that he would have radiation for five days to try and reduce the tumor as well as make him more comfortable.

I would send a text message every day and check-in. Sometimes, I would get an answer, sometimes not, which was always concerning. But he operated differently than I did and didn't always answer immediately. I was getting a little anxious, to say the least, that I wasn't being told everything.

One evening, I texted Charlie and asked if he had eaten any dinner, as he didn't have much of an appetite. He said he cooked himself something to eat as Ann had gone to bed because she wasn't feeling well. His message read, "I hope she isn't internalizing all that is going on, I know it's harder on the caregiver sometimes." I had to agree that she probably was, but I didn't write this as I didn't want to make him feel bad or make it sound like I didn't understand, or maybe that I understood better than he realized I did.

I texted Ann the next day and asked how she was, "I'm fine, just sitting here playing games on my tablet." It seemed all was back to normal there for now. I wanted to offer her encouragement and mostly "courage." I had to gather my courage every day with all that was going on here, and I hoped she had some as well, the next few months were going to be difficult for her.

I wanted desperately to go see Charlie and Ann. Charlie's birthday would be in August, and I wanted to be there. I asked Bill, "What would you think if I went to see Charlie in August?" His flat answer, "No!" I wasn't surprised, but my feelings were a bit hurt. We were also worried about the Covid upsurge, and he didn't want me to fly. Bill never told me "No" to anything, but I knew he would not like being at home with a caregiver for a few days. I had to abandon my idea for my trip.

I sat down to send an email to Charlie to tell him I couldn't come for his birthday after all. He said he understood, and it was okay because the doctor told him, "You aren't going to die right away." I had no response to this. What a harsh way to tell someone they will be okay for a while, but only for a while.

Charlie began some different type types of treatments. Chemo was not an option for him. He began an infusion of a medication every three weeks to try and give him some time and quality of life. I then got another text message from him that said the treatment wasn't that bad, but he wasn't sure if cancer or COPD was killing him. He had both, and they were progressing fast.

We then had a "fight" basically while texting. The worst way to communicate because it doesn't reflect the emotion behind what you are saying, especially if you are trying to be funny. He quit writing, and then when he finally did, he wrote something hurtful, and it didn't make a whole lot of sense. He told me, "At least I won't die alone, like you will."

I told myself he wasn't feeling well, he didn't mean it, and all would be better soon. I would give him some time to feel better before I wrote back. My niece told me he went to the hospital by ambulance the same day he wrote the terrible message. He must have been in bad shape; and probably doesn't even know what he wrote. I waited until he felt better to write again.

I found these tips for talking to someone when they may be dying within a short time. I think they are worth looking at for anyone who is dealing with death and dying at any time.

Be sure to follow the dying person's lead.

1. Listen for cues the person is ready to talk about dying. The mention of new symptoms, or not being alive for an upcoming event, or being tired of being sick. This might then give you the opportunity to ask, "Do you want to say more about it?" or "I'm not sure what you mean?" When you ask these questions, it is important to then listen and ask more questions to make sure you know what they are referring to. Let the dying take the lead.

2. Be clear that you know the end is near. Some people avoid talking about death until close to the end. It is not a comfortable subject for most people to discuss. It is common that the dying may find love and support when you are open and honest in the conversation. You might ask, "What is it you need from me?" If they can't answer this question, then perhaps the support you offer is being there

and listening, running errands, or helping with housework. "Call me if I can do anything for you," is probably the least supportive thing one can offer, as it forces the dying to then make the call and ask for help. Make it easier on them by showing up and doing some of the tasks that you might see as helpful to the dying and their family.

3. If there are regrets, ask for forgiveness.

    When the final good-bye is inevitable, this is not the time to be bothered about regrets and past hurtful words. You may feel you disappointed the person during their life and want to express your sadness about it. "Please forgive me," will go a long way in expressing the sadness you may be feeling for past transgressions, whatever they might be.

4. Turn it around and express forgiveness for any hard feelings with, "I forgive you."

    There may be deep hurt in your relationship and forgiving the person will let go of anger and any wish to punish the person for hurts you may have experienced during their lifetime.

5. Express thanks for the positive way the person touched your life.

    Acknowledging what the dying may have done in their life and how it affected you. It is as easy as saying "Thank you." It can restore dignity and let the person know they mattered during their life.

6. It's never too late to say, "I love You."

    Said freely and often can take a relationship to a happier level at the end of someone's life.

7. Say "Good-bye" before it's too late.

    Don't wish you had said "good-bye" at the end of a person's life by being afraid to say it while they are still alive. It's a reminder of how important they were to you and can prevent regrets like, "I wish I would have said good-bye and I love you, before they died."

8. Talk with touch.

When words are difficult or no longer heard, touch can often say many of the same things. It tells the person you are there, and they are not alone.

Source: Canadian Virtual Hospice

Since Charlie lived several states away, I would not be able to go to his bedside and repeat any of these ideas. But if I didn't want to have regrets about his death and not being able to see him, I needed to start saying these things now. I could have called, texted, or emailed since I can't visit but, I would have to get my nerve up in case he rebuffed my attempts at reconciliation.

Expressing these things is hard, but the regrets, if you don't say anything, can be harder to live with. This goes way beyond the normal comfort level with death and dying for most people. Practice in front of a mirror or with a friend if you need to but do try and let your dying loved one know that you are there if needed; you love them and will always remember them.

I Can't Do This Anymore

Lesson: Give Me Strength Instead of Fear

I woke up every now and then, well, more frequently than I like to admit, thinking, "I can't do this anymore!" I would get out of bed and try and approach the day slowly and then think, it will be okay, nothing will happen today. I just need to slow down and do what I need to do. This worked quite well until it seemed everything gathered like a storm cloud and dumped on me all at one time.

Bill was coughing more and sleeping more, and I could tell what was happening. He was getting worse. His appetite was poor, and he was losing weight. This also meant he was getting weaker, and walking was becoming more of an issue for him. He always used a walker now because a cane was not enough support. One day, he asked me to go buy him a new walker. The one he was using at the time had three wheels, and he wanted one with four, so it was more stable. He felt he was getting weaker and wanted the extra support.

Sometimes he would try and walk across the hall to the bathroom at night and wouldn't make it all the way to the toilet. There would be pee on the floor or the rug. I didn't find this so terrible, I just asked him to tell me when it happened, so I could clean it up so no one or the dog would walk in it. To solve this problem, I got a bedside commode for him, placed it by his side of the bed, and put a urinal in it that he would use when he woke up at night. It had to be emptied every morning, but that was not a big deal. We learned to live with this!

The next day I woke up to a chirping smoke detector. Such an annoying noise. It was Memorial Day weekend, and I thought, "I'll never find anyone to replace the batteries on a Saturday of a holiday weekend." I walked the dog, hoping it would stop while I was gone, knowing that it probably wouldn't.

I then made a call to the handyman we had used in the past to see if he could possibly come to replace the batteries. I left a message on his answering machine. The big problem was our 10-, 12-, and 14-foot ceilings in the house. The ladder was the issue. I would have easily changed the battery if I could have reached the ceiling.

I called one of my neighbors down the street that I knew had a ladder, and she brought it down. She was able to reach the two smoke detectors on the 10- and 12-foot ceilings, but not the one on the 14-foot ceiling. So, she ran off to check with other neighbors to see if anyone had a taller ladder. She went to houses where I had never met the owners. She was on a mission. I wanted her to stop. Nothing I said mattered. For an hour, we scoured the neighborhood, or I should say she did.

My neighbor continued to get everyone involved and eventually found a gentleman with a ladder around the corner and down the street. He drove it to the house and brought it in. It weighed a ton. We couldn't seem to get it set up, and he got his fingers smashed trying to get it to work. I got him some ice, but he left, but I knew he was in pain. He walked to his house and left his truck in front of my house. I said at this point, "That's it, I'm calling a halt to this. I can't be injuring my neighbors with this crazy smoke detector thing."

So, we carried the ladder out to the truck and went to check on the man with the injured finger. Before we got to his house, his wife came stomping down the sidewalk toward us with venom in her eyes. I knew we were going to get chewed out. He came out and called her back, so I didn't have to listen to her "yell" at us, or me, since it was my house with the smoke detector problem.

He came back to my house to move his truck with the ladder in it. I asked him how his hand was, he said, "I've got an ice pack on it." I told him, "I'm sorry you got hurt." He drove off. He hasn't spoken to me since.

I had enough! Two hours have gone by, I'm just about in tears, and this stuff normally doesn't upset me. It's just a pain in the behind. Bill hasn't had breakfast. He got out of bed when the "ladder search" was going on, and the first thing he said to me is, "We've got a chirping smoke detector." "Ha, no kidding, Bill," I wanted to say to him, but I stopped took a breath, and tried to keep moving and solve the problem. By now, it's 10:45 a.m., and I had gotten a message the handyman would arrive about 1:00 p.m. "Thank you, so much." I texted, "We can manage until then." I got a smiley face back.

I got Bill some breakfast and finally, go brush my teeth

and take care of the day's chores. I was planning to get Bill's New York Times at the grocery store like I do every Saturday, but he tells me, "Oh no, you don't have to go now. It's okay." I felt terrible about this because reading his newspapers is the highlight of his day.

Bill went back in the bathroom to finish cleaning up, I went to help him, I came out of the bedroom after a few minutes and stopped in the hallway, listened, and by God, the smoke detector had quit chirping. The silence was wonderful, but I would still have the battery replaced when the handyman came, as it was the final one of the four smoke detectors in the house, and I wasn't going through this day again if I could help it. It wasn't even noon yet, and it already felt like an eighteen-hour workday.

If a chirping smoke detector could bring me to tears, I needed to do some more work on myself and my anxiety. I "had to get a grip," as they say. "One day at a time, take deep breaths and don't let the neighbor take over making a small issue into a neighborhood disaster." I had let everything that was going on cloud my thinking, making a simple smoke detector's chirping control my anxiety.

I had an app on my phone that sent me little messages during the day telling me to "Breathe," or asked me how I was doing, giving me choices like I'm anxious, tired, restless, stressed, or sad. I usually checked in with the app when it came, and it would send me a little message back. On this day it told me, "Leave yesterday behind in your thoughts, you don't know what will happen tomorrow, so worrying does no good, be concerned only with today and it will be gone before you know it."

A week later, I heard another chirp in the hall when I

woke up. It didn't seem to be coming from the smoke detectors. The handyman who helped me the week before told me, "It's more often the CO_2 monitors chirping, not the smoke detectors" Ahh, I remembered this and went to check the two CO_2 monitors in the house, one was in the bedroom and the other in the hall by the front door. It was the one by the door that was merrily chirping away.

I had bought batteries during the week, so I put in a new one, and the chirping stopped. Hallelujah! I took a few deep breaths and walked the dog to begin my day as I normally would. The day continued, and it turned out to be a much quieter Saturday with no drama.

At great times of frustration or anxiousness, our instinct is to react rather than respond. When we react, as I did with the smoke detector and everything else that was going on, it makes things worse. By screaming and getting mad, it just makes our mind and bodies more stressed. When we choose to focus and calm down and take deep breaths, we make a conscious decision to create a better outcome.

I needed to work on this. I know when my voice gets out of control, the dog will run and hide in her crate, that's not good. If the dog senses it, then it must be pretty obvious. I need to tell myself, "I can do this." Saying "I can't." will not help the situation and leads to more anxiety.

The Bloody Nose

Lesson: There is Always Something to be Thankful For

On December 28th, 2019, we woke up to a grey, cloudy day after the Christmas holiday. It was a Saturday and would just be a normal quiet day for us. I would maybe put some Christmas decorations away and probably sew or quilt like I normally would. The holidays were usually quiet at our house.

Normally we didn't have much company over the holidays. Except for this year, I changed our normal holiday tradition by inviting Bill's daughters and their families over on Christmas for a bit of champagne and some holiday treats. This had never happened before, hard to believe in over twenty-eight years of marriage, we had never spent a holiday with his kids. Bill had been feeling so poorly for the last six months that I wasn't sure there would ever be another holiday with him for them, so I took a giant leap and invited them over.

We had an enjoyable day and toasted to the New Year. The girls reminisced about Christmas when they were younger, and we enjoyed a lot of laughter and fun, making me feel that I had done the right thing in inviting them. I breathed a big sigh of relief when it went well. The two daughters, one with her daughter and the other with her husband and son, left with smiles on their faces. I was happy I had invited them after an afternoon full of good cheer and warmth.

Just a few days later, this happy Christmas would mean even more as we almost lost Bill to what is unbelievable to me - a bloody nose. I was in the kitchen making some scones for breakfast when I heard him yell, "I need some help in here!" I ran down the hall and found him leaning over the sink in the bathroom with blood pouring out his nose. "Sit down on the toilet, hold the bridge of your nose and I'll get some ice."

He did as I told him, but the blood was still pouring out. I thought "Bill's Pradaxa, won't let his blood clot, this could get bad." Pradaxa is an anticoagulant he takes to prevent strokes due to his atrial fibrillation. I told him to keep pressing on the bridge of his nose, and I got some more towels and ice, but in my mind, I thought, "I will never get him to the hospital if this keeps up." I decided to call 9-1-1 for an ambulance.

I got the dog in her crate, opened the front door, and turned on the flasher. All the houses where we lived had a switch that turned all the outside lights on and made them flash so the emergency personnel could find the address easily.

The fire department arrived first. I had Bill's medications printed out for them, I handed the paper to one of the EMT's and told them his history. One fireman said, "You are good, we should have you on all our calls." I told him, "I was a nurse, I was used to giving a report."

One of the ambulance crew had been at the house before, and he went in the bathroom to check Bill and said, "His nose has stopped bleeding, I don't think you need us." My retort, "You are taking him, I cannot drive and control a bloody nose at the same time." He smirked, I could have slapped him, but he said, "Okay, but I don't think he needs to go by ambulance."

They grudgingly loaded him into the ambulance. I got dressed and got the dog situated, gathered my belongings, got the scones I had been baking out of the oven and turned it off, and started for the hospital. It wasn't even 8:00 a.m., and the day had begun in a whirlwind.

I arrived at the emergency room just as they were getting Bill settled. They had him on the monitor for his heart and the oxygen saturation monitor. His oxygen level was pretty good, but only at about ninety-five. I told the nurses and the doctor that he had been on oxygen for six months and that he should probably have it on while in the emergency room. This fell on deaf ears.

A nurse came in and checked him. His nose was still bleeding, but only a little. He had blood all over his clothes, and I asked, "What happened, you are covered in blood." "My nose let loose again in the ambulance and the guy really wasn't ready for it." I wanted to hunt the ambulance driver down that had said he didn't need to go by ambulance and tell him, "I told you so!" But there were more important things to take care of, and it wouldn't have done any good.

The doctor came in, and I mentioned the oxygen again. He didn't comment, checked Bill, and said he would be back and put some packing in his nose if it didn't stop bleeding soon. It didn't stop. In fact, it got worse and poor Bill couldn't wipe the blood away fast enough, so they attached a little handheld device called a yankauer tip to the suction tubing so he could suction his own nose.

The yankauer is a stiff plastic device with a curve and a small hole that is connected to suction tubing that is usually used to clear mouths and throats of some sort of drainage or saliva. It didn't work, as Bill could not see where the blood was coming from or where to place the end of the device. I took hold of it and sat on the bed by him, and continued to suction all the blood that was pouring from his nose. By now, the blood had run down his neck onto the bed and his clothing; it was really a gruesome sight.

He told the nurses I was a nurse, and so they just walked out of the room and let me take over. It was a busy morning, but I was beginning to feel that they were treating his bloody nose as "just a bloody nose." They didn't start an IV which is protocol when someone is bleeding, and they didn't start him on oxygen as I requested several times. They just left the two of us to deal with the bloody mess. Eventually, the doctor came back in and said he would pack Bill's nose. Finally, something was going to happen, eventually.

A nurse who had not been in the room before came in to check on him, looked for his IV, and there was none. She had a nice friendly chat with him, very cordial, but nothing was being done. I told her about his oxygen use at home, and she said to me, "Why don't you sit down and let us do our job!" I answered, "I'd be happy to, if you were doing your job!" Just then, Bill had a seizure. She told me to leave the room and called for help.

I would not leave, another couple of nurses came in, and I mentioned he used oxygen at home, yet one more time. He came around quickly, and it was determined it was a "hypoxic seizure." The lack of oxygen to his brain made him have a seizure. Well, if you need oxygen, this is one way of telling the nurses, but not the healthiest way. They put an oxygen mask on him that had small holes on the sides so I could continue to suction the blood pouring out his nose.

I wanted to scream at the nurses, "Bill is someone's father, husband and son, he's an important man, but mostly he is a human being, and you are ignoring him." I did not, but oh, I was so close. They finally started an IV and gave him some nausea medication because the blood was now draining down his throat and making him nauseous. He continued to bleed. It was clear this was not "just a bloody nose."

My patience was getting thin, or I should say there was none left. I can only say this, that I could have stamped my feet and made a bigger fuss about them not listening to me. But, would it have made the situation worse or better? I will never know, but they eventually did get the message; Bill was in serious trouble.

This is not the way an ER normally operates, and the head nurse came to apologize to us for all the mishaps. But we were well into later in the day by then, and I couldn't help thinking the damage had already been done.

While this was going on, I texted Bill's oldest daughter and told her we were in the emergency room. We had such a joyful holiday that I wanted her to be aware that her dad was in trouble. Bill prefered I didn't tell his daughter's anything, but I felt it was their right to know they might be losing their dad.

She arrived and brought me a coffee, and we waited to see what was going to happen next. I was still in charge of suctioning his nose. The doctor came back in and finally put some packing in Bill's nose and walked out. We waited to see if it worked, and if it did, we could go home. We didn't wait long, and the bleeding started again. I was back to suctioning the blood before it ran down Bill's face, but he was also swallowing it, and it made him more nauseated.

This went on until about 8:00 p.m. - packing, suctioning, repacking, more suctioning, but he continued to bleed through the packing. A head and neck doctor (once known as ear, nose, and throat doctors), named Doctor Amy, had been called in by now, and she would take over the packing. Finally, it seemed to have stopped, so I thought I could get home for the night. They were going to move Bill to a room where he could be watched closely but be out of the emergency room.

When I got home, the dog was very upset. She looked all over the house for Bill. I finally got her settled down with more food, even though a neighbor had gone in and fed her and let her out while I was gone. After I calmed down, she did as well, as she seemed to sense my emotions, and we both settled down to my comfort food of popcorn and a glass of wine.

The next morning, I thought I was going in to pick Bill up and bring him home, but just as I was getting ready to leave, I got a call from Doctor Amy, who had repeatedly packed Bill's nose several times during the night. She had spent most of the night with him, suctioning and replacing the packing. "It has to be a ruptured artery in his nose, I have to take him to surgery, and I am very doubtful he will survive it because of his lung problems." I gasped, teared up and told her, "I'll be there in 30 minutes. That's as fast as I can get there." She told me, "Go to the ER, I don't think they will have him moved to surgery by the time you get here." "Okay." Was all I could say, and I made a mad dash for the car.

While driving to the hospital, I called Bill's oldest daughter that had spent part of the day with us on Christmas and told her what was happening. She lived closer to the hospital than I did, so I told her to get there as soon as she could. I then called the other daughter and very carefully told her what was happening and where to go see her dad. I did not want to panic her but wanted her to know, "We are in an emergency situation with your dad, you need to get to the hospital as soon as you can." I didn't have time to dumb things down for her, I just wanted her to get to the hospital if she wanted to see her dad, possibly for the last time.

When I got to the ER, Bill told me what happened during the night, "The doctor couldn't stop the bleeding, she kept packing my nose, but it didn't work." "I'm so sorry you should have called me!" I told him. "It's okay, there was nothing you could have done," he said. He started bleeding even more, and I was back in control of using the suction again.

The nurses moved him to surgery with his daughter and me in tow. I haven't told the daughters that he might not survive the surgery. I tried not to give too much information at once, especially if it was bad news.

We got to the operating room holding area, and it was a whirlwind. The nurses checked him in, started another IV, and prepared him for surgery. The doctor came out to tell me what had happened the night before and what she would do in surgery. Because of Bill's respiratory arrest in surgery six months earlier, everyone was very nervous, except for Bill, it seemed.

The anesthesiologist told me one of the big concerns was that they had to turn off Bill's pacemaker to cauterize the ruptured artery in his nose. Bill's heart could then stop beating, or he could have atrial fib again, perhaps causing a blood clot to form in his heart which could then lead to a stroke.

I gave them Bill's entire medical history and helped them get him ready for surgery. Another issue that had to be dealt with was that Bill was a "Do Not Resuscitate." That order had to be rescinded so they could do the surgery, as ethically, a doctor cannot let a person bleed to death without doing something to stop the bleeding. All was moving at a very fast pace. By this time, both daughters have arrived and got to see their dad. We all prayed this was not the last time any of us saw him alive.

In about forty-five minutes, he was ready for surgery, and the girls got to say their good-byes and "I love you's." I stayed with him for as long as I could as I walked by his bed, holding his hand, until we got to the hallway leading to the surgery suite. I couldn't go any further. I gave him a hug and a kiss and told him, "I'll be here when you come out, you are in good hands." He agreed, "I love you," we both said, and off they took him. I only hoped I said enough that he knew how I felt. I took a deep breath and went to go sit with his daughters and wait. I would have rather sat by myself.

The hospital has a system where they give you a number, and you can check an electronic board that will tell you where the patient is. I kept this number handy and watched the board that told me when surgery started and when it ended. We went to get coffee in the cafeteria while I watched the clock. I knew about how long the surgery would take, and I wanted to be back in the surgery waiting room when the doctor came out.

As soon as I saw he was out of surgery, I anxiously waited for the doctor to come out and tell us what had happened. The girls were talking with some of the other people in the waiting area, and I did my best to be pleasant and act like all was well even though I knew we were in a precarious situation.

Doctor Amy came out and said, "Bill is doing just fine. As I suspected he had a ruptured artery in his nose. The obvious symptom being that the bleeding stopped for a while and then started again. The Pradaxa he was on, would not let a clot form, so the artery had to be cauterized."

Packing the nose would have never stopped the bleeding, but they sure tried. I lost count of how many times they put packing in his nose, including little devices that blew up like a balloon inside his nose.

I wanted to hug her, but I asked instead, all in one breath, "How did the surgery go, is he breathing okay now, will he be staying?" She said, "The surgery went well, he did fine. We will keep him overnight, and when he goes home, he cannot be left alone for several days." I said, "I'll take care of him, don't worry."

Bill spent a few hours in the recovery room while I sat with him. The nurses and I watched him closely for breathing, or not breathing for that matter, and he seemed to be doing fine. After about two hours, he was assigned a room.

Today his luck was with him, in more ways than one, it seemed, and he was assigned a private room in pediatrics. There were virtually no patients there, no little kids in the hospital over the holidays! Oh, it was beautiful, quiet, and it was in the same building as maternity, so every time a baby was born, they played Braham's Lullaby over the intercom. How soothing and quiet it was for him to get well and feel better.

After he was settled in bed, I asked Bill, "Are you thirsty or hungry?" He said, "A little thirsty, my throat hurts a little too." "Let me go check with the nurse at the desk, I bet I can get you a surprise." I walked out to the nurse's station and asked, "Since this is pediatrics, do you have Popsicle's?" "We sure do, would you like one too?" I said, "Absolutely!" What a treat at the end of a very stressful day!

Bill spent a quiet night in pediatrics, and I brought him home the next day, which was New Year's Eve. What a way to end the year, but thankfully we ended it together. His oldest daughter called to check on him after we got home and told me, "If you had not been there, my dad would have died." I thanked her with tears in my eyes; it was the nicest thing any of his kids had ever said to me.

My fears of Bill dying would become even greater after this scare. We were lucky, he made it through surgery, and our life would move on, but I was always worried about the next time, and we might not be as fortunate. Little did we know health care would get harder to come by due to the pandemic that was about to close the state down a couple of months later.

Anticipatory Grief

Lesson: Keeping the Scrapbook of Your Life Together in Your Mind

After Bill was given his terminal diagnosis of Idiopathic Pulmonary Fibrosis and the bloody nose scare, I began to worry about the future. It was like "waiting for the other shoe to drop," wondering when and how his death would happen. I didn't want him to suffer and wanted him to be comfortable until the end.

My other great worry, and it seems rather selfish, is what would happen to me? How would I get through all of it on my own? I wondered if this was common. I imagined it was but tried to stop myself from agonizing about the future when I was still dealing with the present. I wasn't very successful at it. I found some interesting facts online about these common feelings for the spouse of someone who has a terminal illness.

I discovered from my research that anticipatory grief, or grief that occurs before death, differs from the grief that happens after a death in that it is seldom discussed with family, friends, or therapists. It seems that it is felt to be socially unacceptable to talk about the grief that occurs in anticipation of an impending death of a loved one. The person could be receiving the support needed to get through this difficult time if they were willing and comfortable discussing their feelings. Anticipatory grief is not reserved just for the survivors. The dying also feel this same strong emotion.

Rather than death alone, this type of grief includes many losses, including the loss of a companion, changing roles in the family, fear of financial changes, and the loss of "what could have been." The loss of time spent together, as well as the memories and dreams of happier times, are all part of anticipatory grief. Grief before death often involves more anger, more loss of emotional control, and atypical grief responses.

This may be related to the difficult place—the "in-between place" people find themselves in when a loved one is dying. A person can feel mixed up inside because they feel they keep failing in the attempt to find the balance between holding on to hope and letting go.

Not everyone experiences anticipatory grief. It's a very individual emotion and may depend on past experiences with death and grief. In some cases, the person may feel a relief that the loved one has passed away and is no longer suffering. For others, very little grief is experienced while a loved one is dying, and in fact, they find they don't allow themselves to grieve at all because it might be construed as giving up hope. Individuals can also experience the grief before the loss even more severely than after the death.

Yet, as painful as the grief is, it can serve as an opportunity for personal growth for the individual who is dying as well as the family. It can provide an opportunity for finding "closure" with family and friends. Reconciling differences, offering forgiveness and a chance to say good-bye. This is the time where conversations can be had that allow the surviving family member a chance to say all the things they might wish they had said after the person dies.

Sometimes, people do not want to visit a dying loved one. They are afraid their grief is so obvious and strong that they don't want the person to see how they are "suffering" as well. Statements like, "I don't want to see them while they are ill, I want to remember them the way they were before they got sick." "I can't handle seeing them sick and watch them suffer." Without understanding that the anticipatory grief they are both suffering could actually be healing if just a brief visit would allow both parties to share their feelings.

Seeing a loved one before they die can help the grieving find meaning in their relationship, even if it was not a good one. For those who are dying, anticipatory grief provides an opportunity for personal growth at the end of life, a way to find meaning and closure. For families, it can be a chance to reconcile differences, as well as grant forgiveness. For both, it is a chance to say good-bye.

Though anticipatory grief doesn't necessarily make the grieving process easier, in some cases, it can make death seem more natural. Seeing a loved one when they are weak and failing and tired might make it a tiny bit easier to say, "It's okay for you to move on to the next place." Giving permission for a loved one to die is also a way of grieving but understanding that the loss is inevitable. It's good for families to talk to their dying loved ones as much as possible and inevitably tell them it's okay to leave. Often the loved one will soon die after the permission from the family has been given.

Anticipatory grief for the loved one and everything the loved one added to a person's life is not a substitute for grief after death. It probably won't shorten the amount of grief a person suffers either. There is no set time span for grief or how someone grieves. Even if the dying individual has been ill for a long time, it won't necessarily prepare you for the actual death. Death is a very individual experience for the dying and their loved ones. It doesn't happen on a schedule, and it doesn't have to be painful. If the dying person is cared for in a loving and nurturing environment, perhaps with hospice involved to ease the pain, death can be a very quiet and humbling experience.

I experienced many deaths when I was a nurse, from babies, kids, young adults, the elderly, and my own family. It was always heartbreaking, but I found that staying with the dying and the family and supporting them in what little way that I could, did make the experience more bearable. I was not a hospice nurse, but I did not fear death, and I managed caring for the dying without difficulty. That does not make me an expert, and when my own loved ones die, I'm not sure how I will act, but I'm hoping my experience can help those that have not experienced death very much, like Bill's children.

These are feelings that one may experience with anticipatory grief. Remember, you may feel them all, or just a few of them, but what you are feeling is not wrong. It is your heart that is breaking. These emotions can ebb and flow, some days will be very difficult, and others will feel like old times and pass without any sadness.

Here are some guidelines to watch for in dealing with anticipatory grief:

- Sadness and tearfulness can rise suddenly and often when you least expect it. Small things, like a walk in a park, passing your favorite restaurant, or watching a TV show you enjoyed together, can remind you of the impending loss.

- Fear of the impending death is mixed with the fear of the changes that will happen once your loved one has passed away. Changes like living alone, having a change in financial security, or perhaps having to move to a smaller residence.

- Anger is a common emotion by both the dying and the survivors of the death. Raging at the unfairness of it all can be common.

- Loneliness is probably one of the more common emotions as life without one's partner, close relative, or friend is hard to adapt to. It may take a lot of time to feel normal again.

- Finding someone you feel comfortable talking with and expressing your emotions is part of healing. It's common to feel that you are boring people when you talk about how you are feeling, so choose your listener carefully.

- Anxiety and hypervigilance are frequently common symptoms when caring for a loved one. This can cause physical symptoms for the caregiver that may seem overwhelming. Sleep difficulty and memory loss can be common.

- Survivors' guilt can happen as one can feel guilty for surviving while their loved one is dying.

- Visualizing the death before it happens. This commonly causes guilt and the feeling that one is not living in the moment but in the future.

You will find more information and coping skills in Elizabeth Kubler-Ross' book called *On Death and Dying*, which was written over fifty years ago. It is still looked at as a premier description of the five stages of grief. Denial, anger, bargaining, depression, and acceptance (DABDA) are the steps one can go through when dealing with death. Not everyone goes through all five stages and not necessarily in that order. Sometimes, a stage can be repeated.

It's important to express your pain and let yourself grieve. Finding a friend or another loved one you can share your feelings openly with is extremely helpful. Maintaining hope and preparing for death at the same time is difficult and being able to express your sadness and cry openly are important ways to get through the grieving process. Some people may find it odd that you are openly grieving before the actual death. These are perhaps not the people to express your emotions with.

Keep in mind that letting go doesn't mean you have to stop loving your loved one—even after they die. During this stage, discovering ways to remember your loved one, such as finding and keeping mementos, looking at old photos, or finding a safe place to store keepsakes, even if it is only memories you store in your heart. This is the beginning of the grieving process that will ease some of the pain that happens later.

Dying is Selfish Business

Lesson: The Long Good-bye

Dying and introspection happening at the same time were a dual reality that I found impossible to ignore when Bill was not doing well. As Bill's poor prognosis and impending death began to reflect on our life, it was getting harder to respond to the living as we had in the past. Bill seemed to be pulling away from everyone he knew, except for a handful of friends and me. As a dying person, he seemed to be concentrating on only one thing - dying. The truth is that nature is selfish and dying is just part of the natural transition as someone ages. You can't avoid it, and sometimes it can even sneak up on you.

The hard reality was difficult for me, that our life was falling apart and changing dramatically when the rest of the world did not seem to notice. In the retirement community we lived in my neighbors often said, "Everyone has something going on." Meaning some illness or family issue affects us all. We are all at an age where we don't seem to be able to escape the reality that "life happens," and with that, so does illness and dying. The thing is nature doesn't care and doesn't stop when our world seems to be falling apart faster than we can count the minutes. Life has its own force, and there is no stopping it.

Where I may have felt that everyone else's life was moving at a different pace than ours, none of this mattered anymore because we only had one thing on our mind in our house, and that was Bill and his illness. I was often, or I should say frequently, asked by neighbors and friends, "How is Bill?" The emphasis was on Bill's health always. My insides were screaming, again very selfish on my part, "I'm not doing so well, but he seems fine today." I only had one neighbor that ever asked, "How are you doing?" when I saw her. I wanted to hug her.

Whether you are the dying or the caregiver, living life to the fullest remains your goal, but somedays it's just too darn hard. When you are so busy that it doesn't seem you have time to take a breath, where does living life to the fullest fit into your day? It may just get a minute or two of your time but knowing that your life can change in a nanosecond may help you try just a little harder to fit life into your life.

Hug your child longer, spend a moment with a sunrise or a sunset, say "I love you." Listen to the last notes of your favorite music on the radio before turning off the car, get out for a walk, or just water your plants and take a walk outside. All will help you seize the moments as they arrive. They are fleeting, so you need to pay attention. Living in the moment takes hard work and practice.

There are many challenges for the dying patient. Some are substantial and overwhelming. A caring physician trained in treating the dying patient may be the source for the best care for the patient. Many physicians are not trained in coping with the dying patient, and this can lead to many miscommunications and discomfort for both the patient and the doctor.

An understanding of the dying patient's experience should help the physician improve their care of the terminally ill. These physicians are often known as palliative care doctors. The doctors specialize in medical care for people living with a serious illness. This care is focused on providing relief from the symptoms and stress of the illness. The goal being to improve the quality of life for the patient and the family. They can assist with the following six challenges that are common to the dying patient:

1. Pain

Pain and the fear of pain often make the patient's behavior change at the end of life. Cancer patients rank "freedom from pain" as one of their goals for care. Even though the fear of pain is there, the elderly are often unwilling to report their pain because they believe it is a normal symptom of aging and that their pain is directly associated with the worsening of their illness.

2. Depression

The presence and severity of clinical depression often correlates with the severity of physical illness and, in some, a progressive inability to get out of bed. A decreased appetite may also suggest major depression. Anxiety commonly co-exists with depression, and it may be driven by fears of helplessness, a loss of control, abandonment, or pain.

3. Coping

Patients with advanced illness face the challenge of coping with their disease daily. While some patients demonstrate optimism, practicality, resourcefulness, awareness, and flexibility, others present with a variety of defensive styles in response to their diagnosis. These defenses can be denial and non-compliance, which can lead to a delay in treatment.

4. Dignity

For dying patients, maintaining dignity is foremost in their care, broadly defined in terms of being worthy of honor, respect, and esteem. For many patients, dignity is directly related to the level of independence retained through the course of illness.

5. The Need for Control

For some terminally ill patients, maintaining a sense of control is a central task of the dying process. This need for control is prominent among patients who request physician-assisted suicide (PAS) in Oregon. These patients were universally described as having strong personalities; they were determined and inflexible, and they wanted to control both the timing and the manner of their deaths.

6. Other Aspects of the Dying Process

Dying patients and their families often must deal with complicated "practical" issues, such as financial problems and legal issues. These seemingly mundane concerns can cause a great deal of distress for dying patients and their families. It's a good idea to take care of the difficult things while the dying can make decisions. Wills, trusts, burial requests, and choosing a grave site can be taken care of while the person is well, so the decisions are not made after the death.

    While nature is selfish, you don't need to be. You might find that your best friend is yourself. You know when you need a hug or when it's time to rest or try to appreciate the moment you are in. You also know when you are at the end of your rope and need to walk away, so things don't blow up and get out of proportion.

There are five regrets the dying often have when it is too late to do anything to change them. There is still time, if you can try and make some small changes now, so your regrets are fewer in the end.

1. *I wish I'd had the courage to live a life true to myself, not the life others expected of me.*

   This seems to be a very common regret when people realize that their life is almost over and look back on it. Many dreams when unfulfilled due to choices they made or did not make. When we are healthy, it's hard to realize that a decision now, which we may only be allowed to make once, can change our life forever. Time may run short, and the chance won't come up again.

2. *I wish I hadn't worked so hard.*

   This regret is more common with men than women. Or it used to be. Since men are often the primary source of income, they regret what they missed while working. Time with children and spouse being the main regret. This is changing now that women are a strong force in the workplace. The working mother who has a child and goes back to work right away may eventually regret the lost time with the child as an infant.

3. *I wish I'd had the courage to express my feelings.*

   Suppressing one's feeling to keep peace with others may result in a mediocre existence and prevent the person from becoming the person they were truly capable of being. Illnesses can result from this, and one may never realize the cause. Mental health is as important as physical health. Bottling up emotions and thoughts is hard on one's psyche.

4. *I wish I had stayed in touch with my friends.*

There are many deep regrets over lost friendships. Getting caught up in one's day-to-day life makes it easy to let friends slip away. Waiting until the end of life is way too late to try and track old friends down.

5. *I wish that I had let myself be happier.*

Many people do not realize that happiness is a choice. We get comfortable in the way we live our lives and don't realize that happiness is easy to come by if we just work at it a little harder and let it in the front door. Fear of change makes people pretend they are happy, but truly they are not. A good laugh and some silliness won't hurt anyone.

Woo, Jennifer A, BA, Maytal, Guy, MD and Stern, Theodore, MD
"Clinical Challenges to the Delivery of End-of-Life Care"
ncbi.nim.nih.gov

When a Good Cry is in Order

Lesson: Tears Are a Normal Way to Express Emotion

Crying is one of life's little outlets that some may think is embarrassing or silly. It's good to cry as it has many benefits you may have never thought of. I don't tend to cry in public or a hospital setting, but I know someday the circumstances will be just right, and I will. It's not that I don't want to cry sometimes, but I just don't have the time. I need to keep moving through the problem or issue and settle it.

When I needed to handle everything for Bill's hospital stays or care at home, that was all I concentrated on. Crying would have just gotten in the way. But was I hurting myself by not letting this emotion come through? I also wondered if Bill could get some relief from a good cry as well.

I decided I needed to investigate the benefits of crying, not that I needed an excuse to cry, but to make sure it was a healthy alternative to handling things instead of the quiet, stoic manner I tended to behave in. I can see a sad movie and cry, but I just can't seem to make it work when I have my job to do; that is taking care of Bill.

I found there are nine ways that crying may benefit your health. Crying is a common human action or reaction, and it can be triggered by many different emotions. But why do humans cry? What is the purpose of a good cry when it comes to soothing a human being in times of distress?

Researchers have found that crying can benefit both your body and your mind, and these benefits begin at birth with a baby's first cry. For older people, crying may have several other benefits, as listed below.

- Crying detoxifies the body.

    There are three different types of tears.

    1. Reflex tears clear debris, like smoke and dust, from your eyes.

    2. Continuous tears lubricate your eyes and help protect them from infection. Continuous tears contain 98 percent water.

    3. Emotional tears contain stress hormones and other toxins. Researchers have theorized that crying flushes these things out of your system.

- Crying helps self-soothe

    Crying may be one of your best mechanisms for soothing yourself. Researchers have found that crying activates the parasympathetic nervous system (PNS). The PNS helps your body rest and digest. The benefits aren't immediate, however. It may take several minutes of shedding tears before you feel the soothing effects of crying.

- Crying dulls pain

  Crying for long periods of time releases oxytocin and endogenous opioids, otherwise known as endorphins. These chemicals known for making us feel good can help ease both physical and emotional pain. Once the endorphins are released, your body may go into somewhat of a numb stage, with oxytocin giving you a sense of calm or well-being.

- Crying improves mood

  Along with helping ease your pain, crying, specifically sobbing, may lift your spirits. When you sob, you take in many quick breaths of cool air. Breathing in cooler air can help to regulate the temperature of your brain. Because a "cool" brain is more comfortable to your body than a "warm" brain. Your mood may improve after sobbing.

- Crying can help get support or a hug.

  Crying is a way to let those around you know you are in need of emotional support or a hug. This is known as supportive crying. From the time you were a baby, crying has been a behavior that told people you needed "care." When you are having a good cry, it is a nonverbal way of saying you are in distress and need help.

- Grief recovery

  Grieving is a process. It involves periods of sorrow, numbness, guilt, and anger. Crying is particularly important during periods of grieving. It may help you process and accept the loss of a loved one. Grieving is a very personal process. If you find that your crying is extreme and it is interfering with your everyday life, it might be time to see your doctor.

- Restoring emotional balance

    Crying doesn't only happen in response to something sad. Sometimes you may cry when you are extremely happy, scared, or stressed. When you cry from happiness or fear, it may be your body's way of helping you recover from experiencing such a strong emotion. This type of crying may help to restore emotional equilibrium.

On average, American women cry 3.5 times each month while American men cry around 1.9 times each month. The averages by country will vary considerably. The average in America is on the higher end of the spectrum. Women in China, for example, only cry about 1.4 times each month, while men in Bulgaria reportedly cry a mere 0.3 times each month.

Tears are a normal way to express emotion. It's amazing that someone counted and averaged how many times a person cries in one month, I'm way behind, so I better get some crying in soon, so I don't ruin the percentages. I make a joke, but this is really a serious way to help you through your grief. The main thing is, if you feel the need to cry, then your body is looking for some relief from anxiety, stress, or sadness, not to mention perhaps happiness. Crying is healthy, and it may help you recover from the sad times in your life faster than holding the tears back.

Aging: The Slow Progression

Lesson: Let Compassion Reign

There is one guarantee in life, and that is you will age, no matter how hard you try not to. Some age with more grace than others, and some age so quickly it's astonishing. Aging can come quickly or slowly; it is not necessarily determined by your age, but the whole dynamics of the life you have lived, and perhaps your relative's lives before you.

Aging isn't just the change from dark hair to grey, or perhaps wrinkled skin that used to be smooth and moist. It is a biological, physiological, environmental, behavioral, and social process. A decline in function and the senses and activities of daily life and increased risk of disease or disability are more accurate definitions of aging.

Aging is the major risk factor for many chronic diseases. Would this mean we want to live a shorter life to avoid these diseases? I believe most would say "NO!" There is always the chance that maybe you won't get one of these chronic illnesses, but you will still age.

There is no single factor to explain aging, and the process can't be slowed. This suggests that if we target aging early on that we can perhaps stop the rate of aging. This would also mean the appearance of aging and possibly the reduction of the diseases related to aging. This would increase what is called "Healthspan." The portion of life spent in good health.

New interventions for the prevention, early detection, diagnosis, and treatment of age-related diseases, disorders, and disabilities must be investigated and researched so we can understand the causes and factors that place people at an increased risk for the aging process. We can't stop aging, but we can slow it down with some general guidelines from all levels of science. Some people are more susceptible to early aging and age-related diseases. But why? Is it genetic, environmental, lifestyle, behavioral, or social factors that initiate the forward march of aging?

It's very clear from the current emphasis on food that diet has a lot to do with the way we live and, therefore, age. Whether we are overweight, exercise or not, eat fats instead of vegetables, smoke, or drink alcohol can determine our early entry into the aging process. Unfortunately, for some, it is too late, and the damage may have already been done. But aging can be slowed down no matter how late you make these changes.

Bill spoke to a palliative care doctor about two years after being diagnosed with Idiopathic Pulmonary Fibrosis. The thought being that the doctor would help us make it easier for Bill to get around, eat, sleep, and remain productive in his remaining life. These are usually the doctors you talk to before hospice is initiated.

Palliative care is an approach that improves the quality of life of patients and their families who are facing problems associated with life-threatening illnesses. I had every hope that this would bring some relief to the day-to-day struggle that Bill seemed to be dealing with. I wasn't sure what I expected, but I thought maybe this doctor had some "magic" that would make things easier here at home.

We had a teleconference call with the doctor and a social worker. Both were very pleasant and well informed about their jobs. The doctor asked, "Bill how are you feeling, what symptoms are you having and what do you think might help you?" Bill answered, "I feel so weak, like I'm slipping away and don't have anything to hang on to." "I cough a lot and choke when I eat sometimes, and I sleep all the time."

Bill's walk had deteriorated quite a bit over the last few years, and I wasn't surprised to hear him say he was weaker. The doctor looked at his medications and suggested he stop two of them because they can both cause weakness. One being the pill to stop acid reflux, which Bill's pulmonologist thought might have caused his pulmonary fibrosis; he could have aspirated food during one of his choking spells.

The other was a drug to stop strokes and heart attacks that was started when he had a TIA. I quickly chimed in. "He was started on that drug when he had the TIA, isn't that dangerous?" The doctor answered, "Yes, he has a ten percent higher risk of having a stroke if he stops taking it." I wanted to yell, "That makes no sense, why would he want to do that?" I ended up saying nothing, knowing I could talk to Bill about it later.

The social worker spoke up and asked, "Have you two ever considered moving to assisted living?" Again, I spoke up and answered, "We have considered it, but I have promised Bill we will stay home as long as I can get help to care for him. I have been to several of the places and the two-bedroom apartments are all upstairs, and that won't work for us!"

Her comment was, "Well, as long as you can afford to stay home." I wanted to ask her, "Do you know the price of assisted living and what many of the places are like?" That was all she had to offer. I was not thrilled with this conversation, as this was not helping us. I backed away, so I could not be seen on the screen anymore.

I let the doctor continue to talk, and he told Bill, "You are not in need of hospice right now, you have a bit longer to live, so that is basically all I can suggest for you, except you should change your diet." Now, I'm wondering what is going on. He told Bill, "Go on a plant-based diet and you won't need the pill to stop the strokes and the heart attacks." My ever kind and sweet Bill says he doesn't know what that means. I'm pretty sure he does. The doctor explained further that he should not eat meats or fats, but he should eat only vegetable-based foods.

I walked away; this was good advice if Bill was younger and had a chance of it helping him. He eats peanut butter and mayonnaise sandwiches and loves a good hot dog or a hamburger, not to mention a steak for dinner. Bill kindly said, "I'll try to eat less meat, thank you doctor." The call ended.

I stopped the two drugs the doctor suggested we discontinue, and in a very short time after stopping the heartburn medication, Bill had heartburn. I emailed his regular doctor, told her what was happening, and she told me to restart the medication. I did, and he was immediately fine.

I had to try to stop worrying about stopping the drug

that prevented strokes. It was Bill's choice to stay off it, and so I would follow his wishes. What was even more worrisome was if I asked Bill about the drug and how he was feeling without it, he didn't remember the doctor told him to stop it.

We were newly initiated to plant-based diets when we hired Bill's second caregiver, who was vegan and ate a plant-based diet and had for most of her life. She was 60 years old and looked 35. This was good evidence to me that the diet worked. She also had some auto-immune diseases, and this diet had kept her off medications. I admired this more than I can say, but I'm not sure we could make these changes completely. Plant-based diets take a lot of work and a lot of planning, and the caregiver seemed to eat only frozen dinners, such as black bean burritos with an avocado every day. Bill would never eat like that.

I thought we should try at least to change our diet, so I bought a simple recipe book and tried some of the recipes. I also bought some plant-based "meat" balls to add to spaghetti sauce. I didn't tell Bill what they were, and he said they were pretty good. I don't think our diet will change completely, but I agree that some changes won't hurt us. Bill will continue to eat bacon, no matter what, I'm afraid.

In this case, Bill changing his diet was not going to stop his aging process; it was probably too late. I've watched him age more in the last five years than I have in the whole time we've been married. Yes, changing his diet may have helped several years ago, but he deserves to be comfortable now too. Idiopathic, as in Idiopathic Pulmonary Fibrosis, means no known cause, so the diet change would not change his diagnosis, and frankly, his living longer with this debilitating disease may not be the most compassionate thing to do for him.

The bottom line really was will any of these changes save Bill? Probably not, and I refuse to let him suffer even if it means giving him a vegetable instead of bacon. He deserves to be comfortable in his remaining days, and one must pick and choose what works for themselves. The doctor's advice was just that, advice. Bill will always let me know what he needs or would like to eat.

A palliative care doctor is trained to make patients comfortable in their remaining years, but I am the one taking care of Bill and need to also take care of myself. Doctors can tell you what's best in their opinion, but they aren't the ones living with the illness. Most patients find the right path and live their lives out as gently as possible to the end (Source: www.nia.nih.gov/about/aging-strategic-directions-research/understanding-dynamics-aging).

We Purchased a Niche

Lesson: Planning Ahead is Always a Good Plan

We had never been afraid of talking about death and dying at our house. I think we were being realistic in our knowledge that the end was near for Bill, and we needed to talk about his desires and requests. I decided it was time for this talk and sat down with him at our 3:00 p.m. cocktail time to have a chat about his thoughts and what he would like me to do with his ashes.

We had already set up our cremation, but there was never any talk about where the ashes would go. Bill would say, "Just put me in the closet with my parents." This was possible, as we have had his parents together in one lovely box in my closet for almost thirty years. Bill did not want to bury his parents when we were moving to different areas because he didn't want them too far away to visit. The closet was the best answer.

It never bothered me, and I would joke with him on May 1st every year, their anniversary. "Have you wished your parents a Happy Anniversary?" He would laugh and say,

"Yes," or "I'll do it later."

Bill had picked out an urn for himself several years ago. It was gorgeous but very big and has been sitting on a beautiful shelf in our hallway for a very long time. I was more than willing to place his ashes in it and keep it in the house, but what would happen to it after I died? I didn't think his children would take his urn with ashes into their homes, so I began to think we needed another plan.

I took a drive and found a small cemetery right in the heart of town. It was a lovely little place with some old and new headstones, green grass, meaning well-tended, and a little area right in the middle with a gazebo and a columbarium niche. This is a wall with several single compartments that hold a person's cremated remains called "niches." These can also be located inside a mausoleum or columbarium or outside, as these were.

I drove through the remaining part of the cemetery, not really knowing what type of burial site we would want if we were interred there. I decided it was worth investigating to see if Bill would want to place his parent's ashes there now and then ours next to them when the time came for us. I thought this outside setting was beautiful and that his parents would love it, and eventually, we would too.

I found the cemetery website and sent an email asking what I would need to do to check the availability of burial sites. I received a very pleasant return email telling me there were four cemeteries in our area, and I could visit them all and make a choice. I made an appointment for us to go to the office and meet with Peter, who managed all the cemeteries. His office was located at the newer cemetery in a part of town we had never been to.

We found the office in the center of the Santa Rosa
Cemetery, but before we parked, I drove around so we could
look at it. It was not as quaint as the one I liked but well
cared for and new. Bill did not like it as well as the older one
in town either, called the First Street Cemetery. We went
inside and met Peter, who would tell us everything we
needed to know about burying someone in one of the
cemeteries.

Peter explained that there were four cemeteries in the
county. "The cemetery on First street that you like, is the
oldest. This one here is called the Santa Rosa Cemetery and
is the newest. There is lots of room for expansion, as you can
see." He pointed to the window, so we looked out and saw
all the room. "The third one is in a small town north of here
and the fourth is called the Cowboy Cemetery. The legend
is that a bunch of cowboys were caught cattle rustling and
were shot on site. They buried them where they fell." We
chuckled at this. What a great story, I would have to go find
this cemetery one day.

We talked about our needs – wanting to inter Bill's
parents with a place for us next to them. We were told about
a new location in the First Street Cemetery that was small
and set up to bury only ashes with a headstone placed over
them. There would be no caskets buried in this area. It was
in the middle of the grounds near the gazebo I had seen on
my drive through several days before.

I got Bill back in the car, and we met the caretaker at the
cemetery so he could show us this new area. It was very
pleasant, with lots of trees and bushes and a place to sit if
one desired. I then saw the niches that were nearby and
asked about them. He explained they were new and that you

can have two people in a niche. We could buy two right next to each other, one for the parents and one for us. Bill wasn't excited about them at first, but he looked around and saw what other people had done with them and decided it was a good idea. The caretaker gave me the numbers of the niches we chose so I could go back to the office and purchase them.

We returned to the office at the Santa Rosa Cemetery and made it known what niches we had decided on. Bill was getting tired with all the driving around and walking and wanted to go home. Peter asked us several questions and told us he would get the paperwork ready for me to come back and sign the next day. I would pay for the niches then. I also had to purchase two metal containers, one for each bag of ashes to go inside the niche, as the cedar box they were in would not fit. I took Bill home and returned the next day, as planned, signed all the paperwork, and wrote the check.

There was some work I needed to do to get Bill's parents buried in our county. Since they did not die in this county, and the cemetery is paid for by local tax money, we would have to pay a fee to bury them here. I would also have to get a permit from the health officer to inter their ashes since they were prepared in another county. I was given a phone number to call, and it turned out to be a very easy process. The next day I drove to the county seat about thirty minutes away and visited the Vital Statistics office to get the proper paperwork completed and then delivered it to the cemetery.

The next big job, which I had no idea I would be taking part in, was the ashes needed to be removed from their current redwood box and placed in the separate smaller containers I purchased that would fit in the niche. I got the cedar box Bob and Alice were currently in out of the closet, put it in the car, and drove to the cemetery to meet Peter so he could open it and move the ashes to the new containers. He said, as he was opening the wooden box, "I'm not worried, they should each be in a separate plastic box or bag, we just have to hope they fit in the new container." Okay, sounds fine to me, I think. I, of course, had no idea what to expect.

He opened the wooden box, which by the way, was very heavy, and there were two plastic bags with "ashes" inside. I put it in quotes because it isn't exactly what I think of as ashes. It looks like bone fragments and bits and pieces of a white substance, not ash. I don't know what to call it. One bag was much fuller than the other, we guessed it had to be Bill's dad since he was a larger man than Bill's mom. This bag was a bit too big for the new box, so we weren't sure it would fit. Peter suggested, "Let's take it outside so we don't get dust all over my office." I agreed it would be a mess, and it was a good idea.

We went outside and slipped Alice's ashes into the new container easily, and then tried to squish Bob's into his without opening the bag. His bag was so much larger that we didn't think it would fit. But with the two of us working, we were able to get the bag in the container without having to open it to pour the ashes in. The bag had a twist tie with an ID tag holding it closed, so bits of fine ash began to come out of the top of the bag as we pushed on it. "Are you okay with this?" He asked me, sounding a little worried. I said, "I'm fine, better me than Bill."

We got the bags of ashes settled, and the new lids installed. I was told the lids cannot be removed without damaging the boxes. He handed them to me and said, "Bring these back with the paperwork when you inter them next month." I thought he was going to keep them, but he had no storage for "ashes," so I put them back in the car, brought them home, and placed them back in the closet until we intered them in the niche. It all went very well, and Bill thanked me profusely for doing all the work. I think he would have cried if he would have had to handle the ashes.

We were set to have a small ceremony for Bill's parents in a couple of weeks. There would not be a service for them. Just us there with the caretaker who would open the niche and put the boxes in. I planned to take a few flowers, and we would spend a few minutes in some silent prayers to place them in their new home. As I drove to the cemetery with the ashes in the back of the car, Bill told them, "Mom and Dad, we are taking you to a nice shady place with beautiful lawn and flowers, I'll join you soon." This was heartbreaking. I fought back tears.

Since we weren't having a funeral service because they both had a memorial service when they died, I wanted to find a simple prayer to set them in their new home. Neither they nor we were were deeply religious, so I spent some time looking around on the internet, but then I pulled out my mother's Bible and looked there instead. My mother kept everything from funerals and memorial services for everyone she knew in her Bible.

I found this anonymous poem on the back of one of the cards that was given to my mother at someone's funeral. I thought it was a lovely verse for Bill's parents, and I read it at the internment when they left our home for good and went to their final resting place.

"In Our Hearts"

We thought of you today
But that is nothing new.
We thought about you yesterday.
And days before that too.
We think of you in silence.
We often speak your name.
Now, all we have are memories.
And your picture in a frame.
Your memory is our keepsake.
With which we'll never part.
God has you in his keeping.
We have you in our hearts.

- *Unknown*

We visit them just about every Sunday. I get us both some coffee, and we go sit on the bench right in front of their niche. It's just a short walk for Bill from the car, so he can get there without much trouble. I take a couple of little flowers because they don't have very large vases attached to the nameplates, and Bill will just sit with them for a while. The cemetery has peacocks that roam around while we visit. We recently discovered that peacocks mean immortality, and a lot of cemeteries have them.

Our preplanning, I believe, will make everything easier when we die. Bill has made it known what he wants, and I will, of course, abide by his wishes. Planning a funeral can be very difficult when all around you seems to be crashing down after the death of a loved one. But if you are not ready to think about a funeral or the planning that might be involved, these guidelines might help make it easier for you when the time comes.

Here are seven ideas that might help you as you begin to think about a funeral:

1. Gather all the vital statistics for the deceased and place in a convenient location so it can be handy when it's time for the funeral. Names of all the family members, the work history of the deceased, and military service information. Don't forget marriage certificates, insurance policies, wills, investments, and retirement account information.

2. Determine who will be involved in the service. Many people have a preference as to who would speak at their funeral and where it should be held. This could include pallbearers, readers, singers, and/or music.

3. If you are to have a viewing before the funeral, make these arrangements ahead of time when the funeral is planned. If there is to be an "open" casket, be sure to include what the deceased will be wearing, including glasses, jewelry, and makeup.

4. Allow the individual to choose their final resting place before they pass away and whether they choose cremation as opposed to embalming and burial. This can eliminate a lot of family discussion and upset and can mean less friction between family members when trying to make plans after the person has died.

5. If your loved one would like an obituary in the local newspapers or magazines, have them prepare their own. This can be difficult to ask, but it is a

clear way of letting the person express whether they want an obituary and how they would like it to read.

6. Make payment arrangements to fund the funeral before the death to remove the financial burden from the family and prevent issues between family members over how much to spend and who is paying for the service.

7. Make a list of all family members and friends to notify of the death. With the stress of an impending funeral, it is difficult to remember everyone you would like to notify. You can also give the list to another family member or friend to contact people, so the burden is removed from your many jobs.

Source: Homesteaders Life Company

Of course, you may have your own idea as to how to celebrate your loved one's life with a memorial service or celebration of life after the person has been cremated and or buried. This can be done at any time; there is no hurry. These choices are all personal preferences, and whatever you choose, it is the right decision. Do not be afraid to go against what some people think is the "normal" way to bury your loved one. If your loved one did not want a funeral, then that is the right decision for you and them. Whatever you and your loved one discussed ahead of time will help you with the decision. If you have a plan written down, that will make it even easier.

I attended a memorial service a few years ago at my neighbor's home a year after her husband died. She handed out a beautiful card with her husband's birth date listed as his Sunrise and his death listed as his Sunset. I can't think of a lovelier way to announce the beginning and end of someone's life.

Caregiving 101

Lesson: Stress is a Function of the View we have of the Event, not the Event Itself

I want to offer guidance and steps to try and help you get through the caregiving experience. It's hard, but it's worthwhile, and it is the most loving thing you can do, but you need to take care of yourself as well. I write this after Bill had to go to the emergency room just last night because he quit breathing. He's okay today, and I brought him home to rest, but my day must continue as though nothing happened and I wasn't up most of the night. I need to take care of myself too, so I refer to this information for me to make sure I stay healthy too.

Many people will become caregivers in their lifetime, or on the other hand, may need one. A "caregiver" is anyone who gives basic assistance and cares for someone who might be ill, disabled, or frail. There are a wide variety of tasks done to assist someone in their daily lives. Balancing a checkbook, writing checks, grocery shopping, doctor appointments, giving medication, or helping with eating, bathing, and dressing are all basic caregiving duties. These duties may occur gradually over time or overnight. For the most part, the caregivers are family, friends, and neighbors and do not get paid. This may feel like something that just comes naturally when you love someone and want to help them when they need it, but it can go on for years and take a physical and even financial toll on caregivers and the family.

Many caregivers in the United States care for an adult with cognitive impairment. This person may have difficulty with one or more of the basic functions of their brain, like perception, memory loss, concentration, and reasoning skills. The diagnosis may be slightly different for the patient, but often, the caregivers for any medical issue share common problems and situations, and ultimately strategies.

Cognitive impairment is not only the loss of brain function; it also can affect how a person thinks, acts, or feels. These add to the challenge of communicating with someone with cognitive impairment as an ordinary conversation can become challenging and frustrating with the person who has difficulty remembering from one moment to the next. These folks require special care, including 24-hour supervision, communication techniques, and management of difficult behavior.

You may also be the caregiver for someone who is ill, has been in the hospital and is recovering, in a wheelchair, or has aged beyond their ability to care for themselves. All caregiving situations have some general strategies you may find helpful. I'm also listing some resources for you to get help if you need it when your caregiving has gone beyond your comfort or knowledge level - in other words if you are at your wit's end and don't know what else to do.

1. Establish a baseline of information. If you go to the doctor with your concerns about your loved one, it is helpful to have a more concise time frame for when they started showing symptoms of needing more care. Answering the question, "How long has he/she been forgetting to take their meds?" With, "Oh, I don't know, maybe a month or two." Is not helpful. It would be better to have an answer like, "I noticed once a week, for the last two months he/she forgets their pills at night before bed."

    By keeping closer track of what is going on with your loved one, it can give the doctor or healthcare worker a better guide for helping with the problem and offering advice. Other questions may be, "Do they forget to pay their bills? How long has this gone on?" "Do they eat a normal diet?" "Are they bothering to cook?"

2. Go with your loved one to see their doctor. Get an accurate diagnosis, find out if there is a medication interaction going on, or if what seems like dementia is really Parkinson's or Alzheimer's that have some treatment options available. Don't assume they are just aging, and nothing can be done for them. A confirmed diagnosis is helpful in planning for the future and determining treatment options.

    If there has been a surgery or a stay in the hospital, get all the information you can on what an expected recovery time might be, what the nurses and therapists did in the hospital as far as helping the patient get well, such as physical therapy. Have a plan of action when your loved one comes home from the hospital.

3. Talk to doctors, health care and social service providers, or people with similar circumstances to get some help.

Education is powerful when you know what is going on and what is expected in their recovery. Read books or pamphlets the doctor may have about the disease or illness. Store all your information in a notebook, so you can refer to it when needed and take it with you to doctor or therapy appointments.

4. Determine what your loved one's needs are as far as physical help or help with daily activities like cooking, cleaning, shopping, dressing, eating, and bathing. Consider changing the normal times they do things so you can be there or when someone else is available to be there. Bathing in the evening, instead of the morning, for instance. Preparing small meals to put in the freezer to be cooked later, if they can use a microwave or oven.

    - Place notes on cabinets reminding them where the dishes or silverware are located.

    - Do the shopping or banking for them so they can be at home and resting instead of leaving the house.

    - Manage medications by using pill containers marked with the days and times of the week.

    - Determine if they need any safety equipment at home, like walkers or canes.

    - Install handles in the shower or bathroom to prevent falls.

5. Make an outline of all the care needs your loved one has. This can help formulate a plan if professional help is needed, and a care plan must be made, so an outside caregiver has the best opportunity of helping where it's

needed. Telling a caregiver, "My husband falls a lot, so you have to watch him, is not as helpful or specific enough to get the best care for your loved one. It would be more helpful to tell them, "My husband needs help getting out of a chair, uses a walker and cannot stand in the shower without help."

These plans are always subject to change, either adding or subtracting required needs for the patient. Be open to these changes. Have a backup plan if a caregiver other than yourself gets sick or can't help you on a scheduled day.

6. Get a full and accurate look at finances. This is always difficult to ask if you have not been involved with them from the start. Find out about long-term care policies that may have been paid for, current obligations as far as house and car payments. What are the expenses for running the house?

    You might consider getting a lawyer or financial planner to help with this as it is easier for them to ask the tough questions and reduce family tensions over money. Make a list of savings and checking accounts, investments, and credit cards. Make sure your name is on all accounts so you can make changes to them if needed. Keep all these records in one place so you can refer to them when the time comes to make changes or move your loved one to another level of care, such as assisted living.

7. Review all legal documents. This can be a delicate subject but will ensure your loved one's final wishes are carried out. You may want to have an attorney bring up these issues and oversee the paperwork. This will take the pressure off you and help you be reassured you are legally

prepared for the future.

You will also want to put Social Security numbers, birth and marriage certificates, divorce decrees, property settlements, military records, income tax returns, wills, trust agreements, and burial arrangements in a safe, easy to access place.

8. Safety proof your home. Make special note of safety hazards when helping an impaired patient. Take special care with the following:

- Fire hazards: stoves, cigarettes, lighters, and matches
- Sharp objects: knives, razors, and sewing needles
- Poisons: medications and hazardous household products
- Remove loose rugs, furniture, and cluttered pathways
- Check lighting at night in hallways
- Lower the water heater temperature to avoid burns
- Cars and driving - do not allow an impaired person to drive
- Remove hoses, tools, gates, uneven pathways outside
- Watch for clothing and footwear that may cause falls
- Mark emergency exits
- If your loved one wanders, place a door alarm on all exits
- Identification bracelet
- Bathroom grab bars and grips

- No rugs in the bathroom or on hardwood floors or use non-skid rugs or mats
- Use paper cups rather than glass
- Supervise food and diet to monitor a healthy intake of food
- Keep emergency phone numbers handy
- Manage all medications
- Supervise alcohol and pain medications to prevent falls

9. Connect with others. Join a support group for social and emotional support as well as sharing practical information and advice. They are also safe and confidential places for caregivers to vent frustrations, share ideas and learn from other caregivers. If you can't leave the house, there are also online support groups that give the opportunity to meet with other caregivers nationwide.

10. Be sure to take care of yourself. This may be the last item on the list, but you will find it to be the most beneficial to your mental health while you are caring for someone else. Caregivers are more at risk for depression, heart disease, high blood pressure, and chronic illness leading to general poor health.

    Here are some guidelines for yourself while you are caring for your loved one:
    - Exercise daily. Even twenty minutes a day will decrease stress, help with sleep, relax muscle tension, and increase mental alertness and energy.
    - Eat healthy meals and snacks. Caregivers often eat on the run, snacking on junk food or skipping

meals. Try to make a habit of eating fruits and vegetables every day.

- Get adequate sleep. Lack of sleep results in exhaustion, fatigue, and low energy, and this all leads to more negative feelings, irritability, sadness, anger, and stress. Ideally, try and get six to eight hours of sleep in a 24-hour period. Arrange for someone to fill in for you during the night if you are up a lot with your loved one.

- Take care of your own medical needs. Get regular medical and dental check-ups. Inform your doctors of your caregiving role and let them know how you are coping. Caregivers are at a high risk of depression, lingering sadness, and apathy.

- Take time for yourself. Recreation of any type is necessary for renewal. Once a week, take time for yourself: read, go out to lunch, or go for a walk, anything that takes you out of the caregiver role.

- Don't forget to breathe. Deep breaths frequently during the day with some meditation is very helpful. There are apps you can put on your phone to help you with both.

- Remember when your life seems like it is surrounded by suffering, assess the situation, learn to live with it, and then embrace it.

The Benefits of Caregiving

Lesson: Putting the Perspective on the Positive

Once you identify yourself as a caregiver, you will find it helpful to look at the benefits of your caregiving role. The National Library of Medicine's resource, MedlinePlus, defines a caregiver as a person who "gives care to someone who needs help taking care of themselves." The recipient could need help for many reasons such as:

- Injury
- Disability
- Chronic Illness
- Advancing Age

This is a simple definition, but for some, the word "caregiver" evokes a variety of meanings, from being a spouse caring for a loved one to a nurse caring for a patient in the hospital. Some would reject the use of the word with statements, like, "I'm not a caregiver, he's, my husband." Many children would protest that taking care of an aging parent is what is expected of them because the person needing care is their parent.

Acknowledging you are a caregiver will give you the benefit of the resources available to you when it comes to getting help with caregiving. Calling yourself a "caregiver" might inspire you to look up ways to make the job easier and more fulfilling instead of thinking of it as "work." It is still hard, but you can ease some of the burdens by thinking of it as a positive experience.

Here is a list of some positive aspects of caregiving.

- *It can give you a sense of purpose*

  When your loved one is ill or at the end of their life, you may find that you have feelings of hopelessness or feel there is nothing you can do to make things better for them. You'll find that by helping to take care of your loved one, it gives your life a new meaning. Service in this manner does not diminish your life, it will enhance it.

- *It can connect you to your humanity*

  The selfless act of caring for someone else will give you a new perspective on your own humanity. It's one of the most loving things you can do.

- *Even If You are Close, You Could Get Closer*

  This is a chance to give back to a loved one. It could be a child thanking a parent for raising them and providing for them or a spouse thanking their loved one for all the good years they spent together. The selfless act of giving all you can to someone else at the end of their life can be very satisfying.

- *This Can be an Opportunity to Resolve Old Feelings*

  When you see someone vulnerable and in need of care,

putting yourself in the caregiver role, can resolve old harsh feelings from the past. You can feel good that you have stepped in and helped when it was necessary.

- *Focus On What is Really Important*

  Caregiving can help you focus on what is important in life. It helps us remember that life is short and old arguments are just not worth bringing up again. You may someday need care yourself; consider this practice.

- *It Can Connect You to a Loved One on a Deeper Level*

  Rather than let caregiving tear you and your loved one apart, try and look at it as a way of refocusing your attention on your loved one's life and what it has meant to you. You may learn you have limitations on what you can do for them, and you may need to do some soul searching to come up with solutions.

- *Satisfaction in Having Direct Conversations*

  The conversations about needed care, death, and dying are very difficult, but you may find that when you approach the subjects with care and concern that you can have these direct conversations, and both you as the caregiver and the recipient of your care may express feelings you never thought you were brave enough to talk about.

- *Teach Future Generations What is Important*

  By caring for someone else, the children that may be involved, whether they be your own, nieces or nephews, and friends, will see that in the future they are better prepared to take on a caregiving role if they see a positive outcome for both the caregiver and the cared for.

Despite all these benefits of your caregiving role, it will be the hardest job you will ever have. The nights can be long and the days short as your loved one may be in bed more than they are out. It can be the loneliest job you will ever have as well, but it can be the most fulfilling.

There are days I will say to you, "I hate this job." It's hard, I get tired, and I wish I didn't have to do it. But that doesn't change anything. I have long talks with myself about continuing to keep Bill comfortable and out of the hospital, yet I wonder who will do this for me?

You may consider assisted living for your loved one, and that will require some research and visits to facilities to check them for staffing, cleanliness, food, level of nursing care, and cost. This will be another hard decision, but hopefully, if you do decide to move your loved one to a care facility, you will have peace of mind that you have made the right decision.

Caregiver Burnout

Lesson: Avoiding Compassion Fatigue

Caregiver burnout is a real and serious problem for those caregivers in it for the long haul. It is a serious issue if you go to bed each night in anguish over the next day's chores and wake up each morning with a feeling of heaviness and a reluctance to get going. Caregivers who feel nothing but dread at the next day's caretaking jobs begin to hate their daily caregiving routines, even if they still love the person for whom they're caring for. There are no longer vacations or long weekends for the caregiver to take a break and care for themselves unless some respite is added to the care plan for the caregiver as well as the recipient.

Without seeking help through counseling or perhaps accepting suggestions for changing the routine of their caregiving day, it is likely these caregivers will struggle unhappily month after month until the day that they simply can no longer physically or emotionally force themselves out of bed anymore.

Emotional outbursts may happen that are aimed at the person they are caring for, which could indicate "compassion fatigue." Expressing emotions that come out as yelling at the person who is ill or disabled can lead to the caregiver being guilt-ridden by losing control of their emotions and saying and doing harmful things they way too often do not mean. The caregiver role can ruin a loving relationship as the burden becomes too much.

These caregivers need to find an alternative means for ensuring their loved one is well cared for so they can take a break. When the caregiver experiences depression and is acting out in uncommon ways, it is at this point that the current care plan or schedule must be reexamined to prevent a toxic environment for both caregiver and recipient. Don't ignore your own exhaustion, eat right, and take your medications as prescribed as well as any vitamins or supplements your doctor recommends.

Most caregivers get thrown into the caregiving position with no experience and no expectation of how long they will be in that role and what they will need to do to keep their loved one safe, fed, warm, and on the correct medications. Caregiving can start out with just the basic needs of helping someone dress or getting them meals, but the role can expand exponentially as someone's illness goes on for perhaps years.

Caregiving is a marathon, not a walk in the park. The family member who accepts this role blindly is like the misguided runner in flip-flops and a skirt with no clue about how far they must run. They are likely to stumble or fall at the beginning of the race because they are ill-prepared. A caregiver stumbling can lead to dire consequences for themselves and the person they are caring for.

Because this marathon may not have an end in sight, it is important that caregiver burden and rising stress levels not be ignored. Marathon runners are constantly assessing their bodies for muscle cramps or strained ligaments that could lead to the end of the race for them. Caregivers, too, need to be on alert for physical symptoms, such as headaches and neck and back pain, and emotional symptoms, such as persistent irritability and hopelessness, either of which could undermine their capacity to give care.

Ignoring burnout can come with some long-term consequences, such as health issues for the caregiver that can lead to their early death or the need for care themselves. The heavy burden of caregiving can gradually overwhelm even the healthiest, most devoted, and best-prepared individuals. This is especially true for sole caregivers who may not have any outside support to fulfill their needs as well as the person being cared for.

Support groups and counseling can be very useful in helping the caregiver cope with the everyday stress of caregiving and caring for themselves as well. We have several groups here in my community, and many are done on the "zoom" format on the computer since it is hard for many caregivers to leave their homes.

So, are you a caregiver? If the title fits, wear it proudly, no matter what your caregiver role is. You might be providing hands-on care or could be an advocate for a vulnerable person. Whatever your job is, you are a caregiver. Be honest with yourself and accept the new relationship with your loved one. Learn to delegate some of the caregiver duties and free up some time for your own emotional support. Focus on the respect you deserve as a caregiver as well as the respect the care recipient deserves.

Dying with dignity is important for all of us, and you as

a caregiver should be proud and feel honored to have assisted your loved one through a gentle and dignified life and eventually a dignified death.

Author's Note

Lesson: When All is Said and Done

As we continue to fight or maneuver our way through the Covid pandemic and try to stay healthy, I constantly remind myself that each day of caring for Bill is a gift. Even when he sleeps most of the day, I know he is quietly snoring his way through the dreams I will never hear about because he won't remember them. Eventually, he will get out of bed and ask for something to eat or wonder where his newspaper is. He will have a smile on his face, walk bent over his walker, and either forget to put his oxygen on or leave his glasses somewhere.

At this point, these few guarantees for the day are enough. We relish our moments together, and even though I feel the need to get away from my caregiver role occasionally, I still come back and put my caregiver hat back on, which is also my cook, laundry, and housecleaning hat. I wonder how long it will go on and if I will be able to meet the responsibilities of a caregiver until the end for Bill.

We've hired several caregivers through different agencies. A few were wonderful, but I also had to fire a few and didn't feel terribly bad about sending someone on their way when they spent an entire four-hour shift on their phone. I'm tired of training caregivers, but if I don't keep trying to find a good one that will stay with us for a while, I will never get to leave the house and feel comfortable leaving Bill alone. I must remember that hiring a caregiver for Bill is taking care of me too.

Writing this book has been a form of "caregiving" for me. Putting my thoughts and feelings into words is a way of healing my breaking heart, knowing Bill will be gone sooner rather than later. I wear my caregiver title with pride and know that I couldn't have done any more to take care of Bill than what I have done.

Be kind to yourself if this role becomes yours. Journaling or writing may be a way of helping you express yourself as well. But, whatever you do, make it yours and make it work for you. You are the keeper of your own mental and physical health.

For your convience here are the chapters related to the **caregiving reference** information:

About Atmosphere Press

Atmosphere Press is an independent, full-service publisher for excellent books in all genres and for all audiences. Learn more about what we do at atmospherepress.com.

We encourage you to check out some of Atmosphere's latest releases, which are available at Amazon.com and via order from your local bookstore:

The Swing: A Muse's Memoir About Keeping the Artist Alive, by Susan Dennis

Possibilities with Parkinson's: A Fresh Look, by Dr. C

Gaining Altitude - Retirement and Beyond, by Rebecca Milliken

Out and Back: Essays on a Family in Motion, by Elizabeth Templeman

Just Be Honest, by Cindy Yates

You Crazy Vegan: Coming Out as a Vegan Intuitive, by Jessica Ang

Detour: Lose Your Way, Find Your Path, by S. Mariah Rose

To B&B or Not to B&B: Deromanticizing the Dream, by Sue Marko

Convergence: The Interconnection of Extraordinary Experiences, by Barbara Mango and Lynn Miller

Sacred Fool, by Nathan Dean Talamantez

My Place in the Spiral, by Rebecca Beardsall

My Eight Dads, by Mark Kirby

About the Author

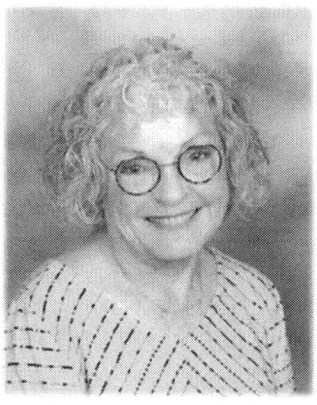

Nancie Wiseman Attwater is a retired critical care nurse, nationally known needlework teacher, author of fourteen books, and a caregiver to her husband Bill. Her nursing education and training as well as compassion for the terminally ill have created this reference guide for caregivers. It is a long and loving look at caring for her husband as he progresses through his illness, many hospitalizations, and entry into hospice care.

She has shared her personal experiences and coping skills to create a book full of down-to-earth guidance when one is faced with the death of a loved one. With humor and empathy she expertly discusses all aspects of the diagnosis of a terminal illness to planning the funeral and dying with dignity all while giving advice on keeping one's own soundness of mind.

Nancie lives in a small community in Northern California with Bill and their dog Grace.

Made in the USA
Columbia, SC
10 July 2022

63086044R00152